A GUIDE
HOMOEOPATHIC

C000002595

A GUIDE
TO
HOMOEOPATHIC
REMEDIES

The Complete Modern Handbook for Home Use

Paul Houghton, RSHom

SOUVENIR PRESS

First published 2000 by
Souvenir Press Ltd.,
43 Great Russell Street, London WC1B 3PA

ISBN 0 285 63557 3

Typeset by Rowland Phototypesetting Ltd.,
Bury St Edmunds, Suffolk

Printed in Great Britain by Biddles Ltd.,
Guildford and King's Lynn.

To A.H.C.

ACKNOWLEDGEMENTS

Major contributions to this project have been made by Shirley Gay, Tony Pinkus and Tessa Harrow.

This book could not have been written without the help and support received from Pamela Houghton and Dr Pam Taraba.

P.H.

CONTENTS

NOTE TO READERS

The aim of this book is to provide information on the uses of homoeopathic remedies in the treatment of relevant conditions. Although every care has been taken to ensure that the advice is accurate and practical, it is not intended to be a guide to self-diagnosis and self-treatment. Where health is concerned—and in particular a serious problem of any kind—it must be stressed that there is no substitute for seeking advice from a qualified medical or homoeopathic practitioner. All persistent symptoms, of whatever nature, may have underlying causes that need, and should not be treated without, professional elucidation and evaluation.

It is therefore very important, if you are considering trying homoeopathic remedies, to consult your practitioner first, and if you are already taking any prescribed medication, do not stop it.

The Publisher makes no representation, express or implied, with regard to the accuracy of the information contained in this book, and legal responsibility or liability cannot be accepted by the Author or the Publisher for any errors or omissions that may be made or for any loss, damage, injury or problems suffered or in any way arising from following the advice offered in these pages.

INTRODUCTION

Which homoeopathic remedy is good for this condition? What is this homoeopathic remedy good for?

These are the most important and frequently asked questions about homoeopathy. The aim of this book is to answer them as fully as possible, for as many remedies and conditions as is practical.

Collecting all the information about a health problem, getting a clear understanding of what is going on and looking for the right remedy are skilful tasks which professional homoeopaths have spent years learning to do. Clearly, this is beyond the ability of untrained individuals. At the same time, the underlying principles are quite simple and there is much that people can do for themselves. Homoeopathy has wonderful healing powers, some of which can only be appreciated by long study and observation of its effects. Yet even experienced homoeopaths are sometimes obliged to work with little more than hunches and the most tentative explanations. This text aims to be clear and frank about the limits of both self-prescribing and professional help with homoeopathy for the conditions covered. It is hoped that this will help you to get the best results out of both.

HOW HOMOEOPATHIC REMEDIES ARE PREPARED

Homoeopathic pharmacy is very simple. The starting point is the juice of the plant which is squeezed out and then mixed with just enough alcohol to preserve it. This is called the mother tincture.

Potentisation

Then the special process of repeated dilution and agitation, called potentisation, begins. The homoeopathic pharmacist takes one drop of mother tincture and adds it to 99 drops of pure alcohol. Then he strikes ('succusses') the vial in which the mixture is contained on a hard surface a few times. The result is potency one.

Next he puts one drop of potency one into another 99 drops of alcohol and succusses again. The result is potency two. And so it goes on. At about potency 12 there is no trace of the original substance left at all, but this is hardly the beginning of the process. Homoeopaths often use remedies in potency 30, 200, one thousand, ten thousand and even one hundred thousand.

Then pills, tablets or granules are coated with the solution, or it is dissolved in dilute alcohol, which can be placed in the mouth. Again the process is very simple. Often the pharmacist just puts a few drops of the potency into a glass vial filled with tablets.

The 'strength' of potencies

In the higher potencies new dimensions of healing power are revealed that were quite invisible before preparation. But it is important to remember that the remedies are only 'stronger' in a special sense. They can only affect someone who has symptoms similar to those that are produced by the remedy. Only then is there the sensitivity in the person to that particular remedy (see p. 5). If someone does not have this sensitivity, the remedy will have just a very subtle effect on them which they probably will not even notice.

Insoluble substances

In the case of remedies made from insoluble substances such as minerals, the first few potencies are made by 'trituration'. One part of the substance is placed in a mortar and 99 parts of milk sugar are added, and the two are ground together thoroughly, to make potency one. Then one part of this mixture is added to another 99 parts of milk sugar and this is ground together, and so on. After the first few stages the same ratio of the powder mixture is dissolved in water and alcohol, and the process proceeds from there.

Different scales

When the dilutions, as described above, are one in a hundred this is known as the centesimal scale which is the most widely used system. In some cases, however, the dilution is made one in ten each time, which is the decimal scale. Then the potencies are known as 6X or 6D and 12X, and so on. Strictly speaking, the centesimal potencies ought to be called 6C and so on, but often the C is omitted and potencies are assumed to be centesimal unless it is specified otherwise.

There is one other system, called the LM scale. LM stands for fifty thousand and the substance is diluted in a ratio of one to fifty thousand at each stage, with many succussions each time. This system is almost always given out in drops or even spoonful doses. It is not so common, but a homoeopath might suggest taking a remedy made this way as it has some advantages. The effect is gentler and more cumulative, rather than the sudden impact that can be the result with centesimal potencies.

HOW DOES HOMOEOPATHY WORK?

Life-energy and matter
Try a simple thought-exercise. Think of a dead body, then of a living person. Compare the two. That which is present in one and absent from the other is what homoeopathy and all systems of medicine are concerned with. Oddly enough, we rarely think about it carefully and there is even some disagreement about what it should be called. Perhaps the best name for it is simply 'Life'.

As you can see, Life is a kind of energy, while the body on its own is inert matter. An essential thing about energy is that in itself it is invisible, we are only made aware of it by observing the effects that it has on matter. On the other hand, the essential thing about matter is that in itself it does nothing, it only moves or changes when energy causes it to do so.

The homoeopathic view of health and illness
From these certainties it is known that *whenever our health changes it is the Life energy that has changed, although the effects on the material body are all that can be observed.*

It is worth stressing this because it is the central point on which all the theory and practice of homoeopathy is based. The only way of telling what has happened to someone when they have become ill is to observe the changes in their body (including the subtle body called mind), simply because this is all that can be observed. But it is known for certain that the cause and beginning of the problem are not in the material body, simply because matter on its own cannot change or do anything. The cause and the real nature of the illness are a change in the Life energy, and it is this change that has to be identified and removed in order to restore the patient to health. The whole business of medicine is how to use medicinal substances in order to achieve this.

There are of course some conditions caused by violent damage to or deformity of the body, when physical intervention is essential. This is the domain of surgery and emergency procedures. Homoeopathy is a system of medicine concerned with the treatment of medical conditions, in the strict sense of that word. The need for surgery and its frequently wonderful results have no bearing on the validity or otherwise of homoeopathy in its own sphere. Medicine clearly has a support role in relation to surgery, and the benefits of homoeopathic medicines during and after surgery are well known.

The work of Samuel Hahnemann

Samuel Hahnemann, the eighteenth-century German doctor who founded homoeopathy, dedicated his life to seeking the best way of using medicinal substances to remove the disturbance in the Life energy which he understood to be the root of illness. He was one of those rare scientists who excel both in experimenting and in reflecting on the results to gain insights into the underlying laws at work in what they observe.

Hahnemann perceived that there is a problem with the usual method of using medicines that have the opposite effect to the symptoms of disease, such as giving preparations that cause diarrhoea to treat constipation, or those that cause coldness to treat fevers. He saw that because of the principle of equal and opposite action and reaction, at first the action of the medicine is to reduce the symptoms, but that then the reaction follows and the symptoms come back, often visibly worse than before. This is why bigger and bigger doses of medicine often have to be given.

He experimented with medicines that had an effect *similar* to the symptoms of the disease, and the results were very pleasing. He conducted many experiments himself and also studied the medical literature available at the time, producing a great body of empirical evidence to support his idea that the best way to remove disease is to give a medicine with symptoms similar to those of the disease.

However, he still faced the problem of how to get the benefits from a medicine without suffering the harmful effects as well. He experimented with diluting the preparations and found that it was easier to control the effects. He persisted in this line and to his own surprise made a remarkable discovery. If he diluted the medicines repeatedly, to the point where no material trace of the substance remained, and vigorously agitated the solution before each dilution, then not only were the harmful effects eliminated and the benefits retained, but also a whole new dimension of medicinal powers was revealed, sometimes in substances that were quite inert in their original form. This way of preparing medicines is known as potentisation.

The result was very surprising, but Hahnemann made many careful experiments and repeatedly confirmed that it was true.

How homoeopathic medicines take effect

For a long time Hahnemann thought that he was still working with the principle of action and reaction, only using it in the opposite way to conventional medicine. He thought that when the homoeopathic remedy was given it had an action like the symptoms of the disease, and that then the equal and opposite reaction happened, which was the opposite of the symptoms, so the patient got better.

Then, near the end of his working life, he perceived a new explanation of how homoeopathic remedies work. He reminded himself again that *whenever our health changes it is the Life energy that has changed, although the effects on the material body are all that can be observed.* And the task of medicine is to remove that change.

He therefore came to this conclusion: Disease is just a state of the Life energy. The effect of a potentised medicine is just a state of the Life energy. If the effect of the medicine is accurately similar to the effect of the disease, then the effect of the medicine takes the place of the disease, which thus ceases to exist. Then the effect of the medicine is exhausted, and the Life energy is left free of both, so long as there is no maintaining cause present to renew the disease.

It is not a matter of action and reaction. Actually, it is more like a simple push: the effect of the medicine displaces the disease in the Life energy.

One might ask, why are the two effects not combined, like two sounds or colours? There is no reason in principle why it should not be like this, but experiments repeatedly suggest that what happens is more like what happens when a big wave displaces a small one.

This is the stage Hahnemann had reached in his understanding by the time he ceased work. His theory is perfectly scientific in the sense that it is the simplest and most complete explanation that has yet been proposed to account for the observed facts, it is rigorously logical, and it is supported by a large body of experience.

The current state of understanding

Since Hahnemann died no substantial progress has been made towards a further understanding of how homoeopathic medicines work and exactly how they should be used in all situations. Luckily he himself had achieved enough to enable his followers to do much good. One reason for this lack of progress is that the final version of Hahnemann's treatise on homoeo-pathic principles was lost for a long time and was unknown to the great homoeopaths of the nineteenth and early twentieth centuries, who shaped the way homoeopathy developed and became established during this period. Even today, versions of the action-reaction theory are pre-sented in many of the schools of homoeopathy. Also, developments in conventional medicine have brought great benefits which any workable theory of homoeopathy must acknowledge and incorporate.

Homoeopaths are acutely aware of the need for progress in this area. At the moment there is some optimism that developments in quantum physics will yield answers, but there is not much enthusiasm for seeking new insights through reflection, along the lines indicated by Hahnemann himself. Exactly how best to proceed is an urgent and fascinating ques-tion which lies outside the scope of this book.

CONSTITUTIONAL TREATMENT

What is constitutional treatment?

We all have our strengths and weaknesses. Often, symptoms appear at our weak spots and to treat them thoroughly it is necessary to consider the whole of which they are a part. Homoeopaths call this constitutional treatment.

It is not the condition that determines which kind of treatment is needed, but the whole situation in which the condition occurs. For example, two people are suffering a pain in the stomach. One patient reports that he cannot remember the last time he had a pain in the stomach and that this one started shortly after he had eaten a large cream cake. Another patient says that she is prone to stomach aches, which tend to be worse in the evening and when she has been worried at work. She has been worried recently, because she has been promoted and given new responsibilities.

The first patient does not need treatment for his constitution, but simply for the excessive ingestion of rich food. In the case of the second patient, a characteristic feature of her metabolism is that symptoms tend to occur at a particular time of day. And this happens when her body-chemistry is affected by certain psychological tensions, which in her case arise from concerns about new responsibilities. The homoeopath will make a careful note of the whole physiological and psychological make-up of the individual, because it is this that is below optimal well-being and needs to be treated. This approach does not arise from a preference for 'holism' for its own sake, but from the hard fact that all the relevant factors in a situation need to be taken into account.

The distinction between acute and constitutional prescribing in homoeopathy is similar to that between acute and chronic disease in conventional medicine. Indeed, homoeopaths sometimes use the word 'chronic' as a synonym for 'constitutional'. The only difference is that the understanding of constitutional types, and the possibility of treating chronic disease on the basis of them, is a particular feature of homoeopathic medicine.

Inevitably, not all conditions fit neatly into exactly one or other of the two categories. They are meant to be broad terms of convenience, not definitions of what is possible or how one must work.

A patient may have symptoms in one system while the rest of his body and mind remains relatively healthy. For this reason homoeopaths study the characteristics of the constitutional types in health as well as disease. The most important of these types have now been so well observed that detailed personality profiles of them have been built up in the homoeopathic reference books, and where appropriate an outline of these profiles is included in the descriptions in the remedy section of this book.

Constitutional remedy finder

The purpose of this section is to find out, if possible, which of the constitutional remedy types might be needed in a particular case. It could be used for yourself, or someone you know well, with their full co-operation.

Constitutional treatment is very often beyond what can be done without professional advice. What is said at the beginning of this book about the limits of self-help does apply particularly to this section. However, in some cases, an individual's constitutional type is quite clear, and as the aim of the book is to enable you to help yourself as far as possible, this section is included to that end.

1 Look through the questions. *Respond only to those for which there is a clear answer*, pass over the others. You will probably find there is an answer to no more than a handful of the questions.
2 When you have been through all the questions, make a note of the remedies listed beside the responses you have made. See which ones have been noted most times and then look up the description of those remedies as given in the remedy section of the book. If there is one that seems to fit the case well, that is the one to try, according to the instructions in the section on the relevant condition.

Which, if any, of the following do you *often* find yourself feeling angry or irritable about?
  People taking advantage (staphisagria)
  Exploitation of the vulnerable (causticum)
  Ingratitude (kali carb, staphisagria)
  Intrusion (anacardium, apis, sepia, staphisagria)
  Idiots (nux vomica, sepia)
  People deliberately ruining things for you (china)
  People who don't respect the rules (kali bich, kali carb)
  People who look down on others (anacardium, staphisagria)
  Stupid objections (aurum, lycopodium)
  People who don't think and won't listen (sulphur)
  The trouble caused by little things that keep going wrong (hepar sulph, nux vomica)
  The things that the people who dislike you do (nitric acid)
  People's attitude (mercurius)

Which, if any, of the following do you *often* have reason to be anxious or afraid about?
  Dogs (carcinosin, china, stramonium, tuberculinum)
  Missing an opportunity for a good time (phosphorus, tuberculinum, medorrhinum)
  Heights (sulphur)
  People misunderstanding your intentions (thuja)
  Big events coming up (argent nit, gelsemium, lycopodium)
  That things are never going to work out for you (psorinum)
  How dirty everything is (syphilinum)
  People who dislike you finding a way to get you (anacardium, mercurius, nitric acid)
  Getting left behind (calc carb)

Going out (gelsemium)
Losing everything (bryonia, psorinum)
Being left all alone (pulsatilla, phosphorus, stramonium)
Bad luck (rhus tox)
Evil (stramonium, psorinum)
Your careful plans not working out (arsen alb)
Loud noises (borax)
People taking what is rightfully yours (veratrum)

Which of the following, if any, particularly apply to the way you feel?
It is difficult to be confident about the best way to respond to things (anacardium, baryta carb, gelsemium, graphities, lycopodium, silica, thuja)
You get bored easily (medorrhinum, tuberculinum)
You sometimes really think that death would be a relief (aurum, natrum sulph, psorinum)
Making decisions is a difficult thing to do (baryta carb, graphities, pulsatilla, silica)
Making decisions is not difficult (lachesis, nux vomica)
It would be fair to say that you are jealous, possessive or territorial (apis, hyoscyamus, lachesis)
You often feel apathetic, indifferent about things (helleborus, opium, phosphoric acid, sepia)

Regarding company, do you:
generally like plenty of company? (argent nit, arsen alb, phosphorus, pulsatilla, stramonium)
often wish you could be alone more? (natrum mur, sepia)

Which of the following, if any, apply to your life?
You are experiencing learning difficulties (baryta carb)
You have the sort of mind that tends to learn things quickly—and perhaps easily forget them (argent nit, ignatia, sulphur)
You learn things quite slowly but may retain them well (calc carb, graphities)
Your life has been dominated by a great loss, disappointment or sadness (aurum, ignatia, natrum mur, phosphoric acid, staphisagria)
You sometimes think you are actually losing touch with reality (argent nit, hyoscyamus, medorrhinum, stramonium)

Your life has been dominated by a very frightening experience (aconite, opium, phosphorus)

Which of the following, if any, are particularly true of you?
You have strong opinions about things (causticum, lachesis, mercurius, veratrum)
You avoid taking sides in things (lycopodium, silica)
You really feel much better when occupied (apis, iodum, lilium tig, sepia)
You really feel better doing nothing in particular (helleborus, sepia, sulphur)
It would be fair to call you a stubborn person (calc carb, silica)
You particularly like to travel (calc phos, carcinosin, mercurius, tuberculinum)
You particularly like to be at home (calc carb)
You like things to be organised and in the right place (arsen alb, carcinosin, nux vomica)
You work best in chaos (sulphur)

To which of the following, if any, are you particularly sensitive?
Beauty (china, carcinosin)
Noise (asarum)
Sufferings of others (calc carb, carcinosin, causticum, ignatia, phosphorus)
Suggestion (argent nit, phosphorus)
Where people are really coming from (sepia)
Danger (stramonium)
Romance (antim crudum)

Which of the following, if any, applies particularly to you?
You cry, laugh and generally show your feelings only with difficulty (lycopodium, natrum mur, natrum sulph, thuja)
You cry, laugh and generally show your feelings easily (phosphorus, pulsatilla)
You are known as someone who talks a lot (hyoscyamus, lachesis, stramonium)
You are known as someone who laughs a lot (cannabis, phosphorus)
You often find yourself in violent situations (anacardium, hepar sulph, hyoscyamus, mercurius, staphisagria, stramonium)

It would be better for everyone if you were not so mild-mannered (cocculus, pulsatilla, silica, staphisagria)

Physically, your build has always been generally:
light/thin (argent nit, arsen alb, calc phos, china, phosphorus, silica, tuberculinum)
heavy/plump (antim crudum, calc carb, graphities, pulsatilla)

Regarding temperature, you are generally the sort of person who:
feels the cold intensely (arsen alb, calc carb, calc phos, china, hepar sulph, kali carb, nux vomica, nitric acid, phosphorus, psorinum, rhus tox, sepia, silica)
finds too much heat unbearable and prefers the cool (argent nit, apis, iodum, lachesis, pulsatilla)
is really sensitive to both heat and cold (mercurius, lycopodium)
cannot stand draughts (kali carb)

Physically, which of the following, if any, do you have or experience often?
Headaches (natrum mur)
Swellings around the eyes (apis, kali carb)
Sinusitis (kali bich)
Flatulence (argent nit, china, lycopodium)
Liver problems (chelidonium)
Recurring chest complaints (calc phos, phosphorus, tuberculinum)
Stress incontinence (causticum)
Infected spots or acne (calc sulph, hepar sulph, kali brom)
Warts (causticum, thuja)
Sleepiness (opium, phosphoric acid)
Chronic fatigue (carcinosin)
Thyroid problems (iodum)
A craving for salty food (natrum mur)

In your case most of the symptoms are on, or began on:
the left side of the body (lachesis)
the right side of the body (lycopodium)

DIRECTIONS FOR USING HOMOEOPATHIC REMEDIES

Where to get homoeopathic remedies
Some of the more common remedies are widely sold in chemists and health food shops. The brands on the market are of perfectly acceptable quality, so there is no reason not to use these if the remedy and the potency required are available. Otherwise remedies have to be obtained from one of the specialist pharmacies, as listed in this book. Almost all of them provide mail-order services.

How to administer the remedies
This is a simple business and many of the directions found in some old books are really not necessary. There is no need to wait half an hour before or after taking the remedy, nor to avoid coffee, aromatherapy oils, perfumes or toothpaste. The key thing is this: the remedy takes effect through the nerves, not via the stomach. Contact is usually made through the nerves in the mouth. So take the remedy and suck or chew it, or let it disperse if it is a drop, rather than just swallowing it whole. Do this when there is nothing else or any residual taste of anything in the mouth. If you have just eaten something with a strong taste, wait five minutes or until the taste has gone. Do not inhale any strong odours for a similar period either side of taking the remedy.

Giving remedies to babies and small children
Use soft tablets or sugar granules that dissolve straight away. These are available from all homoeopathic pharmacies. Otherwise, crush an ordinary tablet between two spoons and put this in the child's mouth.

Treating animals
Look up the appropriate condition and consider the relevant suggestions in exactly the same way as you would with a human patient. When giving the remedy, if the animal tends to resist taking tablets use quick-dissolving remedies. Alternatively, a good way of giving remedies to animals is with drops: put one or two drops on the nose, which they will promptly lick off. Sometimes people resort to disguising remedies in food. This is not ideal, but usually works anyway.

The common potencies

The most widely used potencies are mother tincture, 6X, 6, 12, 30, 200, 1M, 10M. If it is appropriate to move to a higher potency, it is usually to the next one in that order. Throughout the text the appropriate potency to get is suggested.

REGIMES: HOW OFTEN TO TAKE THE REMEDY

This is a slightly complex question because the answer depends on the reaction to the previous dose. Strictly speaking the rule is to give the remedy and observe the effect. If it does not work it was the wrong remedy—think again. If it does work, do nothing as long as the improvement lasts. When it stops, repeat the remedy.

In practice it can be difficult to decide exactly what to do, so homoeopaths often give their patients directions such as those described below. In the section on conditions, which regime is appropriate is indicated throughout.

NOTE: In all cases it is assumed that medical investigations and treatment are being sought where appropriate without delay. If you are unsure whether or not to seek medical advice, then you should.

Regime A: One dose three times daily for ten days.

If the remedy does not work at all, stop: it was not the right remedy. Consider another remedy or see a homoeopath.

If at any point the symptoms disappear completely, stop. Repeat only if they return.

If there is some improvement, keep taking the remedy so long as improvement continues.

When there is no longer any further improvement, stop after there has been no change for five days and consider whether another remedy is now needed.

If the symptoms improve but come back quickly, or if improvement ceases to progress but the same remedy still seems to be needed, a higher potency may help more (see common potencies, above).

At this stage you have established that homoeopathy could help a lot and it may be strongly advisable to see a homoeopath for specific advice.

Regime A1: One dose three times daily for five days. Otherwise, as Regime A.

Regime A2: One dose daily for ten days. Otherwise as Regime A.

Regime A3: One dose twice daily for five days. Otherwise as Regime A.

Regime B: Take the remedy when the symptoms occur, once every four hours.

If nothing has happened after two days, stop: it was not the right remedy. Consider another remedy or consult a homoeopath.

If there is improvement, proceed according to Regime A.

Regime B1: One dose every hour for three hours, then one every four hours until symptoms disappear or change.

If they disappear, give no further remedies. If they change, choose another remedy according to the new symptoms. If there has been no improvement after two days, stop because it was not the right remedy. Consider another remedy or consult a homoeopath.

If there is improvement, proceed according to Regime A.

Regime B2: As regime B1, except that if there has been no improvement after twelve hours, stop.

Regime B3: As regime B1, except that if there has been no improvement after 24 hours, stop.

Regime C: One dose daily for three days. Try to forget about it for three weeks, then assess what the response has been.

If there has been no change, it was not the right remedy. Consider another remedy or consult the homoeopath.

If there has been an improvement, do nothing until the improvement stops. If the improvement stops or symptoms start to come back, the remedy may be repeated. If there is no response to that, either a higher strength or a different remedy is now needed.

At this stage it has been established that homoeopathy could help a lot and it may be very advisable to see a homoeopath for specific advice.

Regime D: One dose every hour for three doses. If there is improvement, proceed as Regime B above. If there is no improvement, seek medical advice or consult a homoeopath.

Regime E: Five drops in a little water before each meal. Stop with improvement; start again only if the improvement halts. Stop after three weeks if there has been no change.

Regime E1: Five drops in a little water before each meal. Stop if there is a clear improvement; start again only when symptoms reappear. Stop after three months if there has been no change.

Regime E2: Five drops in a little water before each meal. Stop if there is a clear improvement; start again only if the improvement ceases. Stop after six weeks if there has been no change.

Regime E3: Five drops in a little water before each meal. Stop with improvement; start again only if the improvement ceases. Stop after five days if there has been no change and consider another remedy or consult a homoeopath.

Regime E4: Ten drops in a little warm water on retiring. Repeat every 45 minutes for up to three doses unless you fall asleep meanwhile.

Regime E5: Ten drops in a little water before each meal. Stop if there is a clear improvement; start again only if the improvement ceases. Stop after six weeks if there has been no change.

Regime F: Twice daily for one week, then once a week for up to two months.

If there is no change after two months, stop: it was not the right remedy. Consider something else or consult a homoeopath.

If at any point the symptoms disappear completely, stop.

If symptoms partially improve, continue until they have completely disappeared or improvement stops.

If at any point the symptoms change, reconsider which remedy is now needed.

Regime F1: Daily for two months, otherwise as Regime F.

Regime F2: Twice daily for one month, otherwise as Regime F.

Regime F3: Weekly for two months.

Regime F4: Twice daily for three months. Then reconsider if the need still exists. If so, repeat.

Regime F5: Daily while travelling, starting two days before departure.

Regime F6: Twice daily for two months, otherwise as Regime F.

Regime F7: Twice daily for one week, then once a week for up to one month. Otherwise, as Regime F.

Regime G: One dose every 15 minutes until medical help arrives.

Regime H: Three times daily until healed.

Regime H1: Three times daily for two weeks.

Regime H2: Three times daily, plus one more dose immediately at the beginning of each hot flush.

Regime H3: One dose 12-24 hours before the operation. After the operation, three times daily for seven days, and then once daily until healed.

Regime H4: One at night before going to bed and another immediately if a cramp occurs.

Regime H5: One at night before going to bed. Repeat at 45-minute intervals for up to three doses unless you fall asleep meanwhile. On waking during the night, take another dose, and repeat at the same intervals.

Regime H6: Once every four hours. Start on take-off and continue until you are able to get a full night's sleep after the journey has finished.

Regime I: Once every 15 minutes for three doses.

Regime J: Put two drops in an eyebath of water and bathe each eye twice daily.

Regime K: Three doses in 24 hours.

Regime K1: Three doses in one day (morning, noon, night), once a week. Start one week before departure and continue for one week after returning.

Regime L: Three times daily until symptoms change or clear up.

Regime M: Apply cream to the affected area three times daily, and once more after bathing, until relieved.

Regime N: Dilute five drops in 30ml (three dessertspoonfuls) of water and apply to the affected area three times daily and again after bathing, until relieved or healed.

Regime N1: One drop of the tincture or oil applied directly to the area, twice daily, until resolved, for up to two months.

Regime N2: One drop of the tincture or oil applied directly to the area, once an hour for three hours and then three times daily until healed.

Regime N3: After washing the hair, apply 1-2 drops to patches of alopecia or 5-10 drops to the head as a whole, and rub in for 2-3 minutes, then rinse out.

Regime N4: After washing the hair, apply 5–10ml of the tincture to the hair. Use fingers and a comb to make sure tincture is applied to all the hair and scalp. Rinse out after 15 minutes. Repeat daily until lice have gone (once may be enough).

Regime N5: After brushing the teeth, add a few drops of the tincture to the brush and use the brush to gently massage the gums, brushing always down the gums to the teeth. Twice daily.

Regime P: One dose daily starting ten days before the due date.

Regime Q: One dose every half-hour when needed.

Conditions A–Z

ABDOMINAL PAIN
(Also see Bowels and Colon Problems, Constipation, Flatulence)

Pain in lower right abdomen, or around the umbilicus, suspected appendicitis: *bryonia 200*, Regime G.

Pain, perhaps from overindulgence; with irritable mood in tense, active individuals; perhaps worse before stool; generally worse moving around; perhaps better for warmth: *nux vomica 30*, Regime B1.

Pain with much wind, pain better if wind passed; chilly and lethargic, but wanting fresh air: *carbo veg 30*, Regime B1.

Pain worse on the right side, worse in the late afternoon, with flatulence; worse when anxious: *lycopodium 30*, Regime B1.

Abdominal pain, some relief when moving around and with fresh air; placid or weepy or needy mood; worse after rich, heavy food; especially during pregnancy: *pulsatilla 30*, Regime B1.

Occasional episodes of sharp, cutting pains, perhaps during diarrhoea; better for doubling up and pressing, or lying on the abdomen; perhaps from or after anger: *colocynth 30*, Regime B1.

Pain before or while passing stool; perhaps with diarrhoea or itching of the anus; in warm-blooded individuals: *sulphur 30*, Regime B1.

Constitutional treatment

Recurrent abdominal pain, whether or not it has been diagnosed as diverticulitis, haemorrhoids or any other condition, requires constitutional treatment. See the constitutional remedy finder for suggestions. If a remedy is well-indicated: that remedy potency 30, Regime B1 during attacks, or potency 200, Regime C between them. Otherwise see a homoeopath. Such conditions usually respond well to constitutional treatment, which can avoid the development of more serious problems later on, so in general it is very worthwhile and advisable to see a homoeopath.

ABSCESSES, BOILS, CYSTS

When the area is painful, made worse by pressure on it and perhaps by cold things, and especially if the patient is unusually irritable: *hepar sulph 30*, Regime B.

In longer-standing or recurring cases when the pain is less intense but there is still matter that needs to be cleared up: *silica 200*, Regime A.

When it is hard to choose between hepar sulph and silica or neither has worked: *myristica 30*, Regime A.

If there is a green or yellow discharge which is smelly: *mercurius 30*, Regime B.

When the infection is not concentrated in a small area, blood and pus are mixed together, and especially if there are red streaks on the skin around it: *pyrogen 200*, Regime B1.

If generalised blood-poisoning is setting in and there is a fever: *pyrogen 200*, Regime B1.

Constitutional treatment

Long-term tendencies to this kind of problem often respond well to constitutional treatment. *Lachesis, mercurius, silica* and *sulphur* types are prone to them. Consider those remedies as described in the remedy section of this book, and see the constitutional remedy finder for more suggestions. If a remedy is clearly indicated: that remedy potency 30, Regime A during attacks, or potency 200 between them. Otherwise consult a homoeopath.

ACNE, ACNE ROSACEA, INFECTED SPOTS

Painful, pus-filled spots that hurt to the touch: *hepar sulph 30*, Regime A.

Spots that are very slow to come to a head or clear up: *silica 200*, Regime A3.

Spots that itch: *sulphur 30*, Regime A.

Spots that definitely come up or get worse at menstruation: *sepia 30*, Regime B.

If nothing else has worked: *berberis aquifolium 6X*, Regime A.

Local application for spots
Alongside any of the above: *calendula mother tincture*, Regime N1, for individual spots, or Regime N for larger areas.

Constitutional treatment

These problems are often metabolic or hormonal, in which case what is needed is constitutional treatment, to which they often respond well. *Calc sulph, kali brom, silica, staphisagria* and *sulphur* are among the types most prone. Consider them in the remedy section, and see the constitutional remedy finder for more suggestions. If a remedy is clearly indicated: that remedy potency 30, Regime A. Otherwise consult a homoeopath.

ALLERGIES, HAY FEVER, ALLERGIC REACTIONS
(Also see Dermititis; Eye Infections)

Running eyes, burning nose: *allium cepa 30*, Regime B1.
Burning eyes, runny nose: *euphrasia 30*, Regime B1.
Violent sneezing: *sabadilla 30*, Regime B1.
Everything running and burning, feeling very tired: *arsen iod 30*, Regime B1.
Everything streaming, feeling very irritable: *nux vomica 30*, Regime B1.
Allergic reactions with tightness of the chest: *arsen alb 200*, Regime D.
Allergic reactions on the skin or mucus membranes, with red itchy rash: *urtica 30*, Regime B1.
Allergic reactions with spots like stings or blisters: *apis 30*, Regime B1.

The use of allergens to prevent or reduce allergic reactions
One approach that sometimes helps is to take the thing to which one is allergic (the 'allergen'), prepared in the same way as a homoeopathic remedy—for example, *pollens 30, cat hair 30,* or *wheat 30*. Most of the common allergens and many not so common ones are available from specialist homoeopathic pharmacies. Allergens may be used alongside other remedies. Dose: *the allergen 30*, Regime A.

Constitutional treatment

Allergies are a disorder of the immune system and the tendency to them is relieved in a substantial proportion of cases by constitutional treatment. All types can suffer from them; among those most prone are *apis, arsen alb, carcinosin, natrum mur, psorinum* and *tuberculinum*. See them in the remedy section, and consult the constitutional remedy finder for more suggestions. If a remedy is well indicated: that remedy potency 30, Regime B during the allergy season or when in contact with the allergen, and Regime C in between. Otherwise consult a homoeopath, which in general is highly advisable.

ALTITUDE SICKNESS

Coca 30, Regime A, starting if possible one day before the ascent to high altitude.

ANAEMIA

If someone is feeling or is diagnosed anaemic after an acute illness, injury, operation, period or childbirth, during which a lot of blood, diarrhoea or other fluids were lost: *china 30*, Regime A.

Otherwise, to help alongside other treatment: *ferrum protox 6X*, Regime A.

Constitutional treatment

Assuming your diet is adequate, the tendency to anaemia means absorption or metabolism is less than perfect. Constitutional treatment will often help a lot. *Arsen alb, calc carb, china, ferrum met, natrum mur* and *phosphorus* types are prone to the problem. See them in the remedy section and the constitutional remedy finder for more suggestions. If a remedy is well indicated: that remedy potency 30, Regime F2 during periods of anaemia, or potency 200, Regime C between them. Otherwise consult a homoeopath.

ANGER, IRRITABILITY, HATRED

Something has just happened or a memory has been brought to the surface and one is feeling really angry, outraged, indignant, feeling that the world is utterly unjust, contemptible: *staphisagria 200*, Regime A1.

Something has just happened and one is feeling really angry, outraged, indignant; it is a total surprise, nothing like this ever happened before, one could scream with the pain of it: *colocynth 200*, Regime A1.

Anger mixed with grief or severe disappointment about something that has just happened: *ignatia 200*, Regime A1.

Anger mixed with grief or severe disappointment about something that happened more than six weeks ago: *natrum mur 1M*, Regime C.

Anger mixed with intense jealousy: *hyoscyamus 200*, Regime A1.

The pressure is really on and one is feeling uncontrollably impatient and irritable: *nux vomica 30*, Regime B.

Dealing with impossible children or situations is threatening to induce a tantrum of one's own: *chamomilla 200*, Regime B.

Feeling that the world is a complete sham; everyone is out for themselves, all apparent goodness is just a trick; feeling angry and hatred at everyone whether they try to be nice or don't bother; constant desire to curse: *anacardium 200*, Regime C.

Constitutional treatment

A general tendency to anger, intense irritability or feelings of hatred may be much relieved by careful constitutional treatment, whether or not there are any physical symptoms to be treated as well. Consider the *anacardium, lachesis, hepar sulph, mercurius, natrum mur, nitric acid, nux vomica* and *staphisagria* types as described in the remedy section, and see the constitutional remedy finder for more suggestions. If a remedy is well-indicated: that remedy potency 200, Regime C. Otherwise consult a homoeopath. It is difficult to be objective about such feelings of one's own, so in general to see a homoeopath is advisable.

ARTHRITIS AND RHEUMATISM, BURSITIS
(Also see Strains and Sprains)

Stiff, sore, bruised feeling in a joint, short or long term, worse for being touched or lying on anything hard: *arnica 30*, Regime A.

Attacks of intense pain in a joint, when any motion makes the pain much worse: *bryonia 200*, Regime B1.

Pain and stiffness, short or long term, worse first thing in the morning or on beginning to move, better for continued motion, worse in cold damp weather: *rhus tox 30*, Regime A.

Tender, lame feeling, pain remains fairly constant whether moving or still, aggravated by pressure or bearing weight, perhaps knees most affected: *ruta 30*, Regime A.

Pain in joints relieved by cold applications, in people who are otherwise generally chilly; worse for movement, especially in the feet and legs: *ledum 30*, Regime A.

Pain in joints relieved by cold applications, in people who generally do not support heat well; pain better for gentle motion: *pulsatilla 30*, Regime A.

Pain in the joints of the fingers: *caulophyllum 30*, Regime A (and consider *causticum* in the remedy section.)

Constitutional and individualised treatment

If none of the above are appropriate or effective, constitutional treatment might help. Among the types most often affected by rheumatism and arthritis are *calc carb, causticum, kali carb, lycopodium* and *medorrhinum*. Consider them in the remedy section and see the constitutional remedy finder for more suggestions. If a remedy is clearly indicated: that remedy potency 30, Regime F2. Treatment needs to be accurate and sustained to make a real difference in this condition, so to see a homoeopath is advisable.

ASTHMA
(Also see Breathlessness)

Treating asthma attacks

A life-threatening asthma attack is one of those situations in which conventional medicine makes complete sense and is generally much more reliable than anything else. Homoeopathic remedies can be safely and effectively used while waiting for medical assistance in severe cases, or during more moderate episodes.

Attacks that come on suddenly, with anxiety, especially in the middle of the night: *aconite 200*, Regime D or G.

The patient cannot satisfy his or her air-hunger, the skin is cold and clammy, and perhaps going blue: *carbo veg 200*, Regime D or G.

Attacks with rattly breathing or nausea, no thirst, shiny tongue; asthma no better after vomiting: *ipecac 200*, Regime D or G.

Attacks with nausea or actual vomiting; asthma better after vomiting; better for cold drinks: *cuprum met 200*, Regime D or G.

Asthma attacks that come on in unusually damp conditions: *natrum sulph 200*, Regime D or G.

Treating the tendency to get asthma

Conventional medicine responds to long-term asthmatic tendencies with regular use of some of the drugs used in emergencies. Lung tissue is highly sensitive, and repeated use of artificial simulators or steroids has obvious implications. Homoeopathic treatment substantially reduces the tendency to asthma in a significant proportion of cases. The more someone has been using conventional medication, the more skilful and patient treatment will have to be. Among the constitutional types most prone to asthma are *arsen alb*, *phosphorus* and *tuberculinum*. See them in the remedy section and the constitutional remedy finder for more suggestions. If a remedy is well indicated: that remedy potency 200, Regime C. In general, to see a homoeopath is advised.

BACK PAIN, LUMBAGO
(Also see Strains and Sprains)

Pain after lifting or straining the back: *rhus tox 30*, Regime B1.

Chronic lower back pain which is worse in the morning and when first moving after rest: *rhus tox 30*, Regime B.

Intense back pain from injury or during illness, when the pain is made much worse by any movement: *bryonia 200*, Regime D.

Pain in the back during a fever, flu or other acute illness, without the particular aggravation from movement: *nux vomica 30*, Regime B.

Pain from injury or degeneration of the spine: *hypericum 1M*, Regime A3.

Pain after repeated strain to the back, such as years of gardening: *bellis per 30*, Regime A.

Pain after injury to the neck: *natrum sulph 200*, Regime A.

Nagging pain between the shoulder-blades: see Liver Problems.

Pain in the region of the kidneys (lower edge of the rib cage at the back): see Kidney Problems.

Constitutional treatment

Some cases of chronic back pain may be further relieved by constitutional treatment. *Calc carb, kali carb, nux vomica, rhus tox, sepia*
and *sulphur* types are particularly prone to the problem, and either *calc
phos, silica* or *sulphur* is often the constitutional remedy for people
who stoop. If any of those as described in the remedy section fit the
case well: that remedy potency 200, Regime C. Otherwise seeing a
homoeopath is recommended, as only accurate prescribing over a prolonged period will make a real difference. Osteopathy, the Alexander
technique and acupuncture have much to offer in this condition.

BED-WETTING
(Also see Incontinence)

Bed-wetting in children or young adults with no apparent anatomical
   or psychological cause: *equisetum 30*, Regime A2 (taken before going
   to bed).
Bed-wetting in adolescents or young adults with depression and low
   self-esteem: *lac caninum 200*, Regime C.

Constitutional treatment

If the above do not help, constitutional treatment will do so in at least
a significant number of cases, even if there is thought to be an anatomical
or other reason for the problem. *Hyoscyamus, lycopodium, silica* and
pulsatilla children are prone to it. See them in the remedy section and
the constitutional remedy finder for more suggestions. If a remedy is
well indicated: that remedy potency 200, Regime A2 (taken before
going to bed). Otherwise consult a homoeopath.

BELL'S PALSY

If the condition has just come on, following a shock or exposure to
   severe cold: *aconite 200*, Regime B1.
The left side of the face affected, especially if brought on by strong
   emotions or in sensitive and sympathetic individuals: *causticum 200*,
   Regime B.
Right side of face affected, no obvious cause: *cadmium sulph 30*,
   Regime A.

Constitutional and individualised treatment

If none of the above are appropriate or effective it is highly recommended that you see an experienced homoeopath about this condition as soon as possible.

BITES, ANIMAL

Severe bite that needs stitching or other surgical attention; person bleeding or in shock or both: *arnica 200*, Regime G.

If there is a significant risk of tetanus or other infection: *hypericum 200*, Regime G (may be given between doses of arnica as above).

Otherwise, to promote healing and reduce discomfort: *ledum 30*, Regime A1.

Local application
Mixture of *hypericum* and *calendula mother tincture*, Regime N2 on individual bites, or Regime N if there is a large area to cover.

BITES AND STINGS, INSECTS

Severe reaction to any bite or sting requiring medical attention: *apis 200*, Regime G.

Bee, wasp or other bites or stings, if the area is red, swollen, perhaps tight as if full of fluid; stinging or itchy, made worse by heat and a bit better by cool; if there is an allergic reaction to insect bites with such symptoms: *apis 30*, Regime B1.

Any other bee, wasp, mosquito or other bites or stings: *ledum 30*, Regime B1.

Local application
Mixture of *hypericum* and *calendula mother tincture*, Regime N2, on individual bites or stings, or Regime N if there is a larger area to cover.

Prevention
In a surprising number of cases it has been reported that the following has substantially reduced the tendency to get bitten by mosquitos, midges and other insects: *caladium 30*, Regime F5.

BLOOD PRESSURE, HIGH (HYPERTENSION)
(Also see Circulation Problems; Heart Conditions; Obesity)

High blood pressure, some irregularity of the heart beat, otherwise reasonably well: *lycopus mother tincture*, Regime E2.

High blood pressure, suspected thickening of the arteries, otherwise reasonably well: *crataegus mother tincture*, Regime E1.

High blood pressure, otherwise reasonably well, few other symptoms: *spartium scop mother tincture*, Regime E2.

Sudden rise in blood pressure after shock or strong emotions: *coffea 200*, Regime C.

Constitutional treatment

Apart from the suggestions above, high blood pressure usually requires constitutional treatment, taking into account the metabolic conditions and mental and nervous tension that are very often its immediate cause. In some cases one of the above remedies may be used alongside or in alternation with constitutional remedies. Any constitutional type could suffer high blood pressure; see the constitutional remedy finder for suggestions. If a remedy is clearly indicated: that remedy potency 30, Regime F. In general it is advisable to consult a homoeopath.

Why different systems of medicine say different things about blood pressure

Looking at someone as a whole, it is clear that the pressure of the blood being pumped out by the heart into arteries is normally the amount that the body needs according to its condition and activity. If blood pressure is reduced for long periods, either by chemically blocking the signals from the body or by stopping the kidneys from reabsorbing fluid, or by any other medical methods, then the natural processes in the body will adjust as far as possible to make up the required blood supplies. Otherwise blood flow to certain parts becomes inadequate and symptoms like coldness of the hands and feet, giddiness and impotence, which are common among patients being treated for high blood pressure, begin to occur.

High blood pressure clearly has its dangers, and medical intervention is effective in reducing it. However the disadvantages of doing so are evident. Medical practitioners generally conform closely to common codes of practice, but there are as yet no rigorously scientific formulae within any system of medicine to guide us in exactly when and how it is best to interfere with the body's self-regulating mechanisms. It is important to follow the best available advice on these matters.

The founder of homoeopathy, Dr Samuel Hahnemann, taught that, in the treatment of all medical conditions, speculation is to be avoided as far as possible and that we should concern ourselves only with the deviations from health that are clearly visible to our senses. This answers in principle the question of how and when to treat high blood pressure. High blood pressure with no symptoms cannot be observed; the implication is that there is nothing to guide us to the required medicine and nothing to justify intervention in the first place. If there is nervous tension or obesity or chest pain or breathlessness or anything else, these are observable symptoms and it is these that are to be treated. It is on this basis that the best homoeopathic treatment can proceed, and for this reason it is especially highly recommended that constitutional treatment is sought if one has been diagnosed as having high blood pressure.

BLOOD PRESSURE, LOW (HYPOTENSION)

Remedies for short-term low blood pressure
If occasionally feeling faint or giddy, particularly when rising (postural hypotension) after a period of illness or severe stress: *cocculus 30*, Regime B.
After injury or loss of blood: see Anaemia.

Treatment of long-term low blood pressure

Someone may be diagnosed as having low blood pressure after complaining of repeated faintness, giddiness, coldness of the hands and feet, impotence or fatigue. These are what the homoeopath would try to correct in the first place, and if treatment was successful, it is likely that the blood pressure would adjust as well. Treatment would be constitutional. Among the types prone to conditions associated with low blood pressure are *china*, *natrum mur*, *sepia* and *phosphorus*. Consider them in the remedy section, and see the constitutional remedy finder for more suggestions. If a remedy is clearly indicated: that remedy potency 30, Regime F. In general it is advisable to consult a homoeopath.

BONE DEGENERATION, OSTEOPOROSIS

Specific remedy
Many cases will respond well to: *calc phos 6X*, Regime F4.

Constitutional treatment

The homoeopathic approach is to improve metabolism and absorbtion generally through constitutional treatment, whether or not the condition is associated with menopause, advancing age or any other factors. *Calc phos, silica* and *calc carb* constitutional types are prone to the problem, if any of them as described in the remedy section of this book seem appropriate: that remedy potency 12 Regime F4. Otherwise consult a homoeopath.

BONE FRACTURES

When the break has just happened, while waiting for medical aid: *arnica 200*, Regime G.
If medical aid is delayed and the pain is particularly severe when the part is moved: *bryonia 200*, Regime G.
To speed up the healing of the bone once it is correctly aligned: *symphytum 30*, Regime H.
Following complex fractures, bone grafts or fractures in people suffering from loss of bone density: *calc phos 6X* and *symphytum 30*, both Regime H.

Constitutional treatment

A chronic tendency to easy fractures may respond to constitutional treatment. See Bone Degeneration, above.

BONE SPURS

To disperse painful bone spurs, such as on the soles of the feet: *hecla lava 12*, Regime F6.

BOWELS AND COLON PROBLEMS
(Chronic constipation or diarrhoea, irritable bowel, spastic colon, diverticulitis, colitis)

Short term relief of symptoms
Whatever the diagnosis, according to which symptoms are actually causing the most discomfort, see the sections on Abdominal Pain, Constipation, Diarrhoea, Flatulence, Piles or Rectal Bleeding for suggestions on remedies for short-term relief of symptoms.

Constitutional treatment

The best way of relieving these conditions, and of avoiding the development of more serious problems, is constitutional treatment to which they generally respond well. Any of the remedies suggested in the sections mentioned above could be needed. See also the constitutional remedy finder. If a remedy is well indicated: that remedy potency 30 during attacks, or potency 200 between them. Otherwise see a homoeopath. In general this is worthwhile and advisable in such conditions.

BREAST-FEEDING PROBLEMS
(Also see Mastitis)

Pain on feeding
If any touch or motion of the breast makes the pain much worse: *bryonia 30*, Regime B1.
If the mother feels weepy and in need of support: *pulsatilla 30*, Regime B1.
If pain goes to the opposite breast: *borax 30*, Regime B1.
Any cases other than those that closely fit one of the above: *phytolacca 30*, Regime B1.

Cracked nipples
First thing try: *phytolacca 30*, Regime B1.
When the cracks are particularly painful: *graphities 30*, Regime B1.
Stubborn cases, where pain in the whole breast is worse when feeding: *silica 30*, Regime A1.
Local application, alongside any of the above: *calendula cream*, Regime M, between feeds.

Too little milk
If the mother feels tearful and in need of support; also hot and wanting lots of open air: *pulsatilla 30*, Regime A.
Otherwise: *urtica urens 30*, Regime A.

Too much milk
Breasts still full and become inflamed on weaning: see Mastitis.
To reduce the flow of milk: *urtica urens 6*, Regime A. (May be given alongside any of the remedies for mastitis.)

BREATHLESSNESS, DYSPNOEA
(Also see Allergies; Asthma; Heart Conditions)

Breathlessness with fear, about something specific: *aconite 200*, Regime B1.
Breathlessness with anxiety without a particular cause: *arsen alb 30*, Regime B1.
From strong emotions: *ignatia 200*, Regime B1.
In stuffy conditions: *pulsatilla 30*, Regime B1.
With a loose cough: *antim tart 30*, Regime B1.
With weakness and tiredness: *carbo veg 30*, Regime B1.

Constitutional treatment

Recurrent bouts of breathlessness need constitutional treatment, taking into account all the factors involved. See the constitutional remedy finder for suggestions. If a remedy is clearly indicated: that remedy potency 30, Regime B1. Otherwise consult a homoeopath.

BRUISING
(Also see Operations)

Severe bruising after an injury or operation, in otherwise reasonably healthy people, for the first ten days after the event: *arnica 200*, Regime A.
After the first week, and in other cases: *arnica 30*, Regime H.
A black eye that is not responding well to arnica: *ledum 30*, Regime A.
An old bruise that is not responding well to arnica: *sulphuric acid 30*, Regime A.

Easy bruising

Long-term tendencies to easy bruising may respond to constitutional treatment. *Lachesis, phosphorus*, and *sepia* are among the types prone to this problem. See them in the remedy section and the constitutional remedy finder for more suggestions. If a remedy is well indicated: that remedy potency 30, Regime F. Otherwise consult a homoeopath. To make a real difference the remedy would have to be carefully chosen and taken for a sustained period, so it is generally advisable to see a homoeopath.

BURNS AND SCALDS

If medical attention is needed: *arnica 200*, Regime G.

If medical attention is needed and the person is shocked: *aconite 200*, Regime G.

Cases not requiring medical attention: *arnica 30*, Regime I, followed by *cantharis* as below.

After the initial shock is over, to relieve pain: *cantharis 30*, Regime A, and *urtica cream*, Regime M, or *urtica tincture*, Regime N.

Burns not healing properly more than three weeks after the event: *causticum 30*, Regime A.

Pains or other effects, such as distress or impaired use of the injured part, which persist for more than six weeks after the burn: *causticum 200*, Regime C.

Local applications

After the pain has subsided and any blistering has gone, to heal the wound and minimise scarring: *calendula 30*, Regime H, and *calendula and hypericum cream*, Regime M, or *tincture*, Regime N.

BURPING, BELCHING, ERUCTATIONS

Burping after a heavy meal or a binge, with stomach ache or constipation, or a desire to burp but inability to do so satisfactorily; irritable mood: *nux vomica 30*, Regime B.

Burping or trapped wind, with bloating and heaviness or lassitude, perhaps after a big meal or a binge: *carbo veg 30*, Regime B.

After a rich, fatty meal, with strong desire for fresh air, perhaps feeling sorry for oneself: *pulsatilla 30*, Regime B.

From nerves before a big event or with that kind of feeling, generally hot and restless: *argent nit 30*, Regime B.

Symptoms tend to come on in the late afternoon, with bloating or discomfort particularly on the right side of the abdomen: *lycopodium 30*, Regime B.

With bloating or trapped wind, in fastidious, anxious, sensitive individuals even if they are careful about diet: *china 30*, Regime B.

Old people burping loudly and uncontrollably: *carbo veg 30*, Regime A.

Constitutional treatment

If none of the above help or the symptoms recur frequently, constitutional treatment is needed. *Agent nit*, *antim crud*, *china*, *lycopodium*, *nux vomica*, *pulsatilla* and *sulphur* types are among those most prone to the problem. Consider them in the remedy section of this book, and see the constitutional remedy finder for more suggestions. If a remedy is clearly indicated: that remedy potency 30, Regime B2 during attacks or potency 200, Regime C between them. Otherwise consult a homoeopath.

CANCER

If at all possible, see an experienced homoeopath before any surgery, chemotherapy or radiotherapy has begun, as the nature of symptoms at this point are particularly significant for homoeopathic treatment. At any stage, however, homoeopathy can help in a significant proportion of cases; often constitutional and specific remedies are used in conjunction.

Some of the most-used specific cancer remedies
Cancer of bones: *symphytum 30*, Regime A.
Brain tumours: *phosphorus 30*, Regime A.
Cervix: *conium 30*, Regime A.
Glands (including breasts, prostate, testes, ovaries): *conium 30*, Regime A.
Intestines and bowels: *hydrastis 30*, Regime A; in advanced cases: *hydrastis mother tincture*, Regime E.
Skin cancers: *arsen alb 30*, Regime A.
Stomach: *condurango 30*, Regime A; in advanced cases: *condurango mother tincture*, Regime E.

Testes: *aurum met 30*, Regime A.
Uterus: *aurum mur nat 30*, Regime A.

Constitutional remedies for cancer

It would be hard to say if any of the constitutional types are more prone to cancer than others. A certain sensitivity, and a tendency to turn blame and criticism in upon themselves more than is constructive or rational, seem to be common features of cancer sufferers. See the constitutional remedy finder for suggestions, but in general it is very strongly advised to see a homoeopath.

CANDIDA ALBICANS
(Also see Thrush, Oral; Vaginal Problems; Flatulence)

Constitutional treatment

The best approach to this condition is constitutional treatment which takes into account the health as a whole and includes both the effects of the candida albicans infection itself and whatever is predisposing the individual to it. See the constitutional remedy finder for suggestions. If a remedy is clearly indicated: that remedy potency 200, Regime C. Otherwise consult a homoeopath.

Specific remedy
It is also possible to take candida albicans itself, prepared like a homoeopathic remedy either alone or sometimes in conjunction with constitutional treatment (see *nosodes*, p. 197). This is not a radical cure, but it does seem to help at least to some extent in a significant number of cases. The usual dose is: *candida albicans 30*, Regime A.

CHICKENPOX

Early stages
The early stages look very much like any other fever or a cold—see those sections. If nothing else is clearly indicated: *ferrum phos 30*, Regime L.

Confirmed cases

When the spots have come up and chickenpox is confirmed, in most cases the best remedy to reduce the fever and minimise discomfort: *rhus tox 30*, Regime L.

If the child is particularly clingy and tearful: *pulsatilla 30*, Regime L.

If the child is particularly bad-tempered and complains of nausea: *antim crud 30*, Regime L.

Local applications

While itching is the main problem: *urtica cream*, Regime M or *urtica tincture*, Regime N.

When the eruptions have begun to fade and are less itchy, to minimise risk of infection or scarring: *hypericum and calendula cream*, Regime M, or *mother tincture*, Regime N.

Prevention

If a child has been in contact with someone with chickenpox, most homoeopaths believe that the best thing is to allow the immune system to proceed naturally. However, if for some reason you wish to do all you can to prevent the illness occurring at this time: *varicella 30*, Regime K (see *nosodes*, p. 197).

CHILBLAINS
(Also see Circulation Problems)

If the pain and itching are worse when the feet are cold: *agaricus 30*, Regime B.

If they are made worse by heat: *pulsatilla 30*, Regime B.

Constitutional treatment

A long-term tendency to chilblains may respond well to constitutional treatment for the underlying circulation problem (see p. 37). The remedies above can be used alongside or in between remedies for the circulation.

CHILDBIRTH

Before the birth
The homoeopathic remedy *caulophyllum* is often taken before to mini-mise the length and discomfort of the birth. Many women have reported being surprised to find how effective it seems to be. Some people think that it would be a good idea for every woman to take some before giving birth; others argue that it is best to take it only during the birth if it is needed, in which case it will work straight away. If you are seeing a homoeopath, or the obstetrician or midwife knows about homoeopathy, follow their advice. Otherwise: *caulophyllum 30*, Regime P.

During the birth
If one of the people attending the birth is knowledgeable about homoe-opathy there are many remedies that might be used. Otherwise the three below are the really important ones to have on hand.

Pain and exhaustion. If at any time the physical and mental strain of it all is too much: *arnica 200*, Regime Q.
Fear. If at any point the mother becomes really frightened: *aconite 200*, Regime Q.
If the labour is progressing slowly, contractions are insufficient and the mother is becoming exhausted: *caulophyllum 200*, Regime Q.

After the birth
(Also see Back Pain, Piles and other specific conditions).
To minimise discomfort and promote healing: *arnica 200*, Regime H.
If there was a big tear or episiotomy or after a caesarean: *staphisagria 200*, Regime H, and *arnica 200*, Regime H.
To apply to the perineum: *hypericum and calendula tincture*, Regime N.
Sleeplessness after childbirth: *coffea 200*, Regime B1, when unsuccess-fully trying to get to sleep.

CHILLS, HYPOTHERMIA

Just after being exposed to severe cold or rain, when the symptoms first start to come on: *aconite 30*, Regime B1.
More than 12 hours after exposure to the cold, if the patient still feels chilled and unable to get warm: *camphor 30*, Regime B1.

If the patient has been severely chilled, feels weak and is blue in parts: *carbo veg 200*, Regime D.

If medical help is required: *carbo veg 200*, Regime G.

CHRONIC FATIGUE, M.E., PVS
(Also see Exhaustion)

Chronic fatigue following an episode of glandular fever or other infectious, debilitating disease, in people who were previously under emotional or nervous strain for a long period: *carcinosin 200*, Regime C.

Constitutional treatment

All the various forms of chronic fatigue, from constant tiredness to M.E., whether they have been diagnosed by laboratory tests or not, usually respond very well to homoeopathic treatment. The diagnosis or label is not important to the homoeopath, just the actual symptoms and the physiological and psychological make-up of the person.

Treatment is constitutional. *Carcinosin* as described above is appropriate in a surprising number of cases. Otherwise, consult the constitutional remedy finder for suggestions and if a remedy is clearly indicated: that remedy potency 200, Regime C. Homoeopathic treatment of these conditions is generally effective, but remedies have to be chosen accurately, taking into account a detailed case-history, so it is recommended that you consult a homoeopath.

CIRCULATION PROBLEMS
(Also see Chilblains; Cramps; Heart Conditions; Obesity; Ulcers)

Remedies specifically for poor circulation
One remedy that will often make a surprising difference for cold extremities or whenever the main problem is simply not enough blood and therefore oxygen getting to the area is: *carbo veg 30*, Regime A. This includes many cases of leg ulcers in the elderly, and Raynaud's syndrome. However, this is usually only a source of short-term relief, not a radical solution.

In a few cases the discomfort or other symptoms are made worse by heat, in which case: *secale 30*, Regime A.

Constitutional treatment

Circulation problems are so much bound up with the overall condition of our bodies that only careful constitutional treatment over a long period is really going to improve things in the long run. Among the types most prone to this sort of problem are *calc carb* (poor circulation in plump, chilly people), *pulsatilla* (plump, warm people), *arsen alb*, *phosphorus*, *lycopodium* (thin-built, chilly people), *lachesis* (lean-built, warm people). See them in the remedy section and the constitutional remedy finder for more suggestions. If a remedy is clearly indicated: that remedy potency 30, Regime F. Otherwise consult a homoeopath, which in general is advisable.

COLD SORES, HERPETIC ERUPTIONS

Cold sores when feeling run-down, sad or irritable. In the case of women, worse around the time of the period; unhappy about the stress of work and family; desire to be alone, but feel better if forced to get up and be active: *sepia 30*, Regime A1.

Cold sores when feeling run down, sad, irritable. Worse during a cold or with a headache, or from the sun; depressed, with a tendency to dwell on what went badly in the past; feel better when alone and quiet: *natrum mur 30*, Regime A1.

If neither of the above apply: *rhus tox 30*, Regime A1.

Constitutional treatment

Long-term tendencies to get cold sores often respond well to constitutional treatment. *Lachesis*, *natrum mur*, *rhus tox* and *sepia* types are among those particularly prone to them. Consider them in the remedy section, and see the constitutional remedy finder for more suggestions. If a remedy is clearly indicated: that remedy potency 30, Regime A1 during an outbreak, or potency 200, Regime C in between. Otherwise consult a homoeopath.

COLDS
(Also see Chills; Influenza; Sinusitis)

Early stages

Symptoms just starting, coming on quickly: *aconite 30*, Regime B1.

Symptoms developing slowly: *ferrum phos 30*, Regime B1.

The patient feels very cold, cannot get warm: *camphor 30*, Regime B1.

Later stages

Clear runny mucous, chilly, irritable, perhaps headache: *nux vomica 30*, Regime B.

Clear runny mucous, chilly, anxious and restless, thirsty: *arsen alb 30*, Regime B.

Discharge from nose making skin sore, symptoms better out of doors: *allium cepa 30*, Regime B.

Thick clear or white mucous, irritable and depressed, perhaps headache, perhaps cold sores: *natrum mur 30*, Regime B.

Thick yellow or green discharge, symptoms better for fresh air, patient wingey or weepy, not thirsty: *pulsatilla 30*, Regime B.

Thick yellow or green discharge, very chilly, irritable: *hepar sulph 30*, Regime B.

Thick or runny discharge, perhaps blood-streaked, better with warmth, patient wants constant company, thirsty: *phosphorus 30*, Regime B.

Thick yellow or green discharge, perhaps blood-streaked, irritable, cold and heat both seem to make things worse; sweaty, clammy skin: *mercurius 30*, Regime B.

Profuse post-nasal drip, none of the above particularly apply: *corallium rub 30*, Regime B.

Constitutional treatment

The tendency to frequently recurring colds often responds well to constitutional treatment. *Baryta carb*, *calc carb*, *calc phos*, *kali carb*, *psorinum* and *tuberculinum* are among the types most predisposed to this problem. See them in the remedy section and the constitutional remedy finder for more suggestions. If a remedy is well indicated: that remedy potency 200, Regime C, between colds. Otherwise see a homoeopath.

COLIC

Classic colic; after feeding, the child curls up, clenches the fists, cries with discomfort: *colocynth 30*, Regime B1.

In a minority of cases the pain causes the child to arch its back rather than curl up. If so: *dioscorea 30*, Regime B1.

As well as having colic the child is particularly bad-tempered and can only be calmed by being constantly carried: *chamomilla 30*, Regime B1.

If the discomfort is obviously caused by trapped wind and relieved when the wind passes: *carbo veg 30*, Regime B1.

Classic colic; after feeding the child curls up, clenches the fists, cries with discomfort, but neither colocynth nor anything else has helped: *mag phos 30*, Regime B1.

If that does not help and no cause for the problem can be identified: *colocynth 200*, Regime B1.

Sometimes when discomfort is obviously caused by trapped wind and relieved when the wind passes, the child is a very young *lycopodium* type. The other things that point towards this remedy are that the symptoms tend to be worse in the later part of the afternoon, the child is more long than plump, and the face tends to wrinkle or frown. If these features are present: *lycopodium 30*, Regime B1.

Constitutional treatment

Stubborn or recurrent cases need constitutional treatment. As noted above, *lycopodium* types are particularly prone to this problem. *Calc carb*, *calc phos* and *sulphur* types might also be affected. See them in the remedy section, and if one is well indicated: that remedy potency 30, Regime B1. Otherwise consult a homoeopath.

COLLAPSE, FAINTING

Sudden collapse, still conscious, perhaps vomiting, anxious and restless but too weak to do anything: *arsen alb 200*, Regime G.

Collapse, breathing weak, skin cold to touch, perhaps cold sweat, blueness, if conscious may be desperate for more air: *carbo veg 200*, Regime G.

Collapse, completely or nearly unconscious, pulse weak, no reactions, laboured or noisy breathing: *opium 200*, Regime G.

Collapse, profuse cold sweat, blueness, patient has been unwell with fever or diarrhoea: *veratrum alb 200*, Regime G.

From shock or fright: *aconite 200*, Regime G (unless *opium* or *carbo veg* as above fit the current condition).

From heat or lack of fresh air: *pulsatilla 200*, Regime B1 (unless *opium* or *carbo veg* as above fit the current condition).

From strong emotions or hysteria: *ignatia 200*, Regime B1 (unless *opium* or *carbo veg* as above fit the current condition).

After collapse and fall on to any part of the body and particularly the head, after regaining consciousness: *arnica 200*, Regime G.

Constitutional treatment

A tendency to repeated episodes of fainting or collapse needs constitutional treatment, taking into account all the factors that are predisposing the individual to this problem. See the constitutional remedy finder for suggestions. If a remedy is clearly indicated: that remedy potency 200, Regime C between attacks. In general, it is highly advisable to consult a homoeopath.

CONFIDENCE LACKING

Short-term difficulties
If a big event is coming up and confidence is unusually lacking, see Fear and Anxiety.

Severe or long-term lack of confidence

This problem may respond well to careful constitutional treatment. *Anacardium*, *baryta carb*, *lycopodium* and *silica* types are particularly prone to debilitating lack of self-confidence. Consider them in the remedy section, and see the constitutional remedy finder for more suggestions. If a remedy is clearly indicated: that remedy potency 200, Regime C. Otherwise consult a homoeopath. It is hard to be objective about such feelings in oneself, so in general seeing a homoeopath is worthwhile and advisable.

CONSTIPATION
(Also see Bowels and Colon Problems; Abdominal Pain)

Urge to go, but unable to do so; irritable mood; perhaps after overindulgence or change of diet: *nux vomica 30*, Regime A1.

Constipation with bloating and gas; tired or lethargic mood: *carbo veg 30*, Regime A1.

No urge, stool very hard: *opium 30*, Regime A1.
Elderly people, with no urge to go: *opium 30*, Regime A1.
No urge, stool large but still soft: *alumina 30*, Regime A1.
Children after eating lots of junk food: *alumina 30*, Regime A1.
If sad or angry about something: *natrum mur 30*, Regime A1.
Nothing else works or is indicated: *hydrastis 30*, Regime A1.

Constitutional treatment

Long-term tendencies to constipation generally respond well to constitutional treatment. *Bryonia, calc carb, graphities, natrum mur, lycopodium, phosphorus, sepia* and *silica* types are among those most prone
to the problem. Consider them as described in the remedy section, and
see the constitutional remedy finder for more suggestions. If a remedy
is clearly indicated: that remedy potency 30, Regime B when the symptoms happen, or potency 200, Regime C in between. Otherwise consult
a homoeopath.

CORNS

Nothing is going to help until rigid, tight-fitting footwear has been
    replaced. Once this has been done: *antim crud 6*, Regime F6.

Local application
Alongside the above: *Ruta mother tincture*, Regime N1 every second
    day, and *tea tree oil* (this is an essential oil, not a homoeopathic
    remedy), Regime N1 on the other days.

COUGHS, BRONCHITIS
(Also see Asthma; Colds; Voice, Lost)

Recent coughs
Dry cough, symptoms just starting: *aconite 30*, Regime B1.
Dry cough, part of an established cold or chest infection, with tickling
    somewhere in the air passages; worse in the morning and at sunset;
    some better for cool drinks; desire for plenty of company: *phosphorus
    30*, Regime B.
Dry cough, part of an established cold or chest infection, with pain in
    the throat or chest when coughing; hot and thirsty for long cool
    drinks; very irritable: *bryonia 30*, Regime B.

Dry tickly cough; comes in violent bouts, worse at night and when lying down; the patient coughs until he or she retches: *drosera 30*, Regime B1.

Whooping cough: *drosera 200*, Regime D.

Dry cough, worse at night and when lying down, with infuriating tickle somewhere in the air passages; the cough is really loud, perhaps croupy: *spongia 30*, Regime B.

Loose cough, lots of rattling but not much coming up, the patient is tired and sleepy: *antim tart 30*, Regime B.

Loose cough, phlegm coming up that is yellow, green or white (in the case of small children who cannot expectorate, there may be discharge of this kind from the nose); symptoms are better in the fresh air; the patient is weepy and clingy: *pulsatilla 30*, Regime B.

Loose cough, phlegm coming up that is yellow, green or white (in the case of small children there may be discharge from the nose); the patient is chilly and cannot stand cold; very bad-tempered, perhaps croupy: *hepar sulph 30*, Regime B.

Loose cough, phlegm coming up that is yellow, green or white but which is tough and sticky and difficult to get up; patient tired and irritable: *kali bich 30*, Regime A1.

Old coughs

A cough left over after an old cold or chest infection that has not gone away after weeks or months, no medical reason: *sulphur 200*, Regime C.

Old person, often coughs, loose cough but does not bring much up, sometimes breathless, generally tired: *antim tart 30*, Regime A.

Chronic bronchitis, phlegm coming up that is yellow, green or white but which is tough and sticky and difficult to get up: *kali bich 30*, Regime A.

Constitutional treatment

Persistent or recurrent coughs need constitutional treatment, to which they generally respond well. See the constitutional remedy finder for suggestions. If a remedy is clearly indicated: that remedy potency 30, Regime Al during attacks, or potency 200, Regime C between them. Otherwise consult a homoeopath.

CRAMPS, MUSCLE
(Also see Circulation Problems)

Cramps in the legs or feet at night: *cuprum met 30*, Regime H4.
Writer's cramp: *mag phos 30*, Regime B3.
Cramping pains in the limbs, which come on in cold or damp weather: *rhus tox 30*, Regime B3.
Cramps in limbs after strenuous work or sport: *mag phos 30*, Regime B3.

Constitutional treatment

If none of the above are appropriate or effective, or cramps recur frequently, constitutional treatment will help in a significant number of cases. Often a circulatory or other problem needs to be taken into account. See the constitutional remedy finder for suggestions. If a remedy is clearly indicated: that remedy potency 30, Regime B1 during episodes, or potency 200, Regime C between them. Otherwise consult a homoeopath.

CUTS, GRAZES, BLEEDING
(Also see Operations)

Cuts that do not require medical attention, once cleaned: *arnica 30*, Regime B1.
Cuts requiring medical attention: *arnica 200*, Regime G.
Severe cuts with heavy bleeding: *arnica 200* and *ipecac 200*, Regime G.
Deep cuts from long, sharp objects such as nails or forks ('puncture wounds'): *arnica 200* and *ledum 200*, Regime B1 or G as above.
Cuts to fingers or toes which are very painful: *arnica 200* as above until bleeding has stopped, then *hypericum 200*, Regime B.
Cuts which ooze blood slowly for a long time: *hamamelis 30*, Regime B (may be given between doses of arnica as above).
Deep cuts that continue to be painful for a long time (including surgical incisions): *staphisagria 200*, Regime A1.
After cuts, once bleeding has stopped, any necessary medical attention is complete and the area has been cleaned; to minimise the possibility of infections and to speed up the healing process: *calendula 30*, Regime A (may be given between doses of any of the remedies above).

Cuts or grazes that get infected while healing: *hepar sulph 30*, Regime B.
If a cut or graze is very slow to heal, repeatedly gets infected, or if foreign
matter remains which cannot be extracted: *silica 30*, Regime A.

Local application for cuts and grazes
Once the area is clean and bleeding has stopped: *calendula and hypericum cream*, Regime M, or *tincture*, Regime N.

CYSTITIS

The word 'cystitis' is commonly used to refer to problems with the
bladder (which is what it really means), the urethra and the kidneys.
This section covers short-term problems in the bladder and urethra
where the main symptoms are frequent or painful urination. Also see
Kidney Problems if appropriate.

Frequent and painful urination, pain worst at the end of urination, few
other symptoms: *sarsaparilla 30*, Regime B.
Frequent urge to urinate, only a little is passed each time, urine passes
in small amounts with intense burning, perhaps traces of blood in
urine: *cantharis 30*, Regime B1.
Cystitis after sexual intercourse, especially first experience or after a
period of sexual inactivity: *staphisagria 30*, Regime A1.
Frequent or painful urination, perhaps during a cold or after a period
of overindulgence; patient irritable, symptoms better for hot applications to the abdomen: *nux vomica 30*, Regime B.
Frequent or painful urination, patient placid or weepy, better moving
around in the fresh air, perhaps in the early stages of pregnancy:
pulsatilla 30, Regime B.
Sudden frequent urging, burning or tingling on passing urine, cloudy
white urine, very painful if urination must be suppressed, urine
escapes if urination delayed: *petroselenium 30*, Regime B.
If there is any pain in the region of the kidneys, or if none of the above
are appropriate: *berberis 30*, Regime B1.

Recurrent cystitis

A tendency to recurrent attacks of cystitis often responds well to constitutional treatment. See the constitutional remedy finder for suggestions.
If a remedy is clearly indicated: that remedy potency 200, Regime C
between attacks. Otherwise consult a homoeopath.

DEPRESSION, SADNESS, MELANCHOLY
(Also see Grief)

Depression about something that happened recently: *ignatia 200*, Regime A3.

Depression about something that happened more than six weeks ago or with no specific object; unable to stop thinking about sad or hurtful events in the past; irritable about little things but unable to do anything about the big ones; cannot or will not weep: *natrum mur 200*, Regime C.

Depression with overwhelming apathy and indifference or mental exhaustion: *phosphoric acid 30*, Regime A.

Depression, hurt, sense of futility, after material loss or redundancy: *aurum met 200*, Regime C.

Depression at time of menstruation or menopause, unable to control temper or tears, longing to be alone: *sepia 200*, Regime A2.

Constant black spirits, sense that the world is irredeemably sad, that trying to change things is futile; melancholy music or old traditions are consoling: *aurum met 200*, Regime A3.

Constitutional treatment

If none of the remedies above are indicated or effective, constitutional treatment is needed for long-term depression. If can afflict any constitutional type, but *anacardium*, *aurum met*, *helleborus*, *natrum mur*, *natrum sulph*, *psorinum*, and *sepia* types are among those particularly prone to it. Consider them as described in the remedy section of this book, and see the constitutional remedy finder for more suggestions. If a remedy is clearly indicated: that remedy potency 200, Regime C. Depression often responds wonderfully to homoeopathic treatment but the remedy must be chosen accurately. As it is particularly difficult to be objective about oneself in these situations, it is strongly recommended that you see a homoeopath.

Suicidal feelings
Such thoughts are the effects of external harmful forces that are attacking us like an illness, and the help of trained specialists is needed. Please seek it. In homoeopathy, *aurum met*, *natrum sulph* and *psorinum* are among the remedies that are particularly relevant.

DERMATITIS, RASHES, URTICARIA
(Also see Bites and Stings; Prickly Heat; Eczema)

Skin reactions from contact

Heat rash: *urtica 30*, Regime B, and *urtica cream*, Regime M, or *urtica mother tincture*, Regime N.

Rash that came up after eating or being in contact with something (particularly a plant); rashes are itchy or burning, bumps like blisters, made worse by heat: *urtica 30*, Regime B1.

Rash that came up after eating or being in contact with something (particularly something chemical); rashes are itchy or burning, desire to scratch but this makes it worse: *sulphur 30*, Regime B1.

Rash that came up after being in contact with a plant; eruptions like poison ivy—large, itchy blisters, itching relieved by heat: *rhus tox 30*, Regime B1.

Severe allergic skin reactions with or without an obvious cause: *apis 200*, Regime D.

Skin reactions to events

If a skin reaction has come up after an event that affected the person strongly, look up that section, for example; Shock, Anger, Fear. If it is in reaction to anger, consider *staphisagria* very carefully; to jealousy or envy: *apis* or *lachesis*; to grief: *ignatia*; to depression or resentment: *natrum mur*. If these are clearly appropriate: that remedy potency 200, Regime A3. Generally, you are strongly advised to see a homoeopath.

Long-term or repeated skin eruptions

Long-term or repeated skin eruptions of any kind require constitutional treatment, taking into account the individual's metabolism and overall health. The skin is the body's front line, so it is necessary to prescribe accurately to raise the level of health further, so that skin conditions can clear up. The types most prone to skin eruptions include *hepar sulph, mercurius, psorinum, silica, staphisagria* and *sulphur*. Consider them in the remedy section, and see the constitutional remedy finder for more suggestions. If a remedy is clearly indicated: that remedy potency 30, Regime A during attacks or potency 200, Regime C in between. For the reasons mentioned above, consulting a homoeopath is strongly recommended.

DIABETES

Specific remedy to reduce blood sugar levels
In the short term, if diabetes has been confirmed and blood sugar levels
   need to be reduced quickly: *syzygium mother tincture*, Regime E.

Constitutional treatment of metabolic conditions

Technically, diabetes means that blood sugar levels are too high because
not enough insulin is being produced by the pancreas. Homoeopaths
and other natural therapists think in terms of a wide range of overlapping
conditions in which the body is not turning food into energy and new
materials efficiently. Often this metabolic disorder is linked in interesting ways to the particular strengths and difficulties that a person is
experiencing on all levels in his or her life.

The management of diabetes with insulin is one of the great triumphs
of modern medicine, but it is not without its disadvantages. The pancreas
quickly loses whatever capacity it still had to regulate these things for
itself and liver, kidney, eye and other problems increasingly arise.

Thorough constitutional treatment early on may help to restore the
balance and avoid these difficulties. *Natrum mur*, *lycopodium* and *sulphur* types are prone to the problem. See them in the remedy section,
and consult the constitutional remedy finder for suggestions. If a remedy
is well indicated: that remedy potency 30, Regime A. In general it is
advisable to consult a homoeopath.

DIARRHOEA
(Also see Bowels and Colon Problems)

An attack of diarrhoea probably caused by eating something unusual
   or spoiled: *arsen alb 30*, Regime B1.
Severe case of diarrhoea, profuse stool expelled with force: *podophyllum
   30*, Regime B1.
Diarrhoea after a binge: *nux vomica 30*, Regime B1.
Spate of diarrhoea with no pain or other symptoms apart from tiredness:
   phosphoric acid 30, Regime B.
Severe case of diarrhoea, signs of generalised food-poisoning such as
   prostration, discoloration of the skin or dizziness: *baptisia 200*,
   Regime D.
Diarrhoea, perhaps with vomiting; the patient is in a weepy, clingy state

of mind, does not want to drink, is hot or wants fresh air, particularly in young children: *pulsatilla 30*, Regime B1.

Diarrhoea, perhaps with vomiting; the patient wants constant company and reassurance, is thirsty and chilly, particularly in young children: *phosphorus 30*, Regime B1.

Diarrhoea from nerves before a big event: *gelsemium 30*, Regime B1.

Constitutional treatment

Recurrent diarrhoea requires constitutional treatment, to which it generally responds well. *Argent nit, arsen alb, china, phosphorus* and *sulphur* types are particularly prone to it. Consider them in the remedy section, and see the constitutional remedy finder for more suggestions. If a remedy is clearly indicated: that remedy potency 30, Regime B during attacks, or potency 200, Regime C in between. Otherwise, see a homoeopath.

If there is a delay before treatment can start, one of the following may help in the meantime.

Recurrent attacks of diarrhoea alternating with constipation, patient chilly and irritable: *nux vomica 30*, Regime B.

Recurrent diarrhoea, worse early morning, patient is either a slightly-built and chilly individual or a more heavily-built and warm person: *sulphur 30*, Regime B1.

Frequent diarrhoea, with much abdominal gas, together with a peculiarly anxious, hurried state of mind: *argent nit 30*, Regime B.

Frequent diarrhoea, with much abdominal gas; the patient is a chilly individual, often anxious, is a perfectionist about things: *china 30*, Regime B.

Recurrent diarrhoea with streaks of blood in the stood; the patient is a slightly-built and sensitive individual: *phosphorus 30*, Regime B.

Recurrent diarrhoea with blood in the stool: *merc corr 30*, Regime B.

EAR PROBLEMS
(Also see Hearing Lost)

Occasional earaches and infections
Pain in the ear comes on suddenly; warm applications feel a bit better; little or no discharge; the patient is anxious and restless; particularly if the episode comes on after exposure to cold: *aconite 30*, Regime B2.

The pain comes on suddenly; the ear is red and throbs, little or no discharge; the patient is hot and flushed, and may be slightly dizzy or delirious; particularly if the right ear is affected: *belladonna 30*, Regime B2.

Severe pain, little or no discharge; the patient cries loudly in pain, only calming down if constantly carried or comforted, there may be a fever or diarrhoea: *chamomilla 30*, Regime B2.

The patient is weepy or clingy or sadly placid; warm applications make the pain worse; yellow or greeny-yellow discharge from ear or nose: *pulsatilla 30*, Regime B2.

Severe pain, worse for touching the area and much worse for cold, better for being wrapped up and especially for warmth; the patient is irritable, if there is a discharge it is smelly: *hepar sulph 30*, Regime B2.

Nothing relieves the pain, everything seems to make it worse; discharge is thin, green or bloody and smelly; patient sweaty and in a foul mood: *mercurius 30*, Regime B2.

Earaches or infections during or after the childhood diseases, particularly measles: *pulsatilla 30*, Regime B2.

Occasional blocked ears, glue ear

Glue ear with little or no pain but perhaps some loss of hearing, a waxy discharge may be visible, few other symptoms: *merc dulc 30*, Regime A1.

Glue ear perhaps with some loss of hearing; patient clingy, weepy or placid; symptoms relieved in the open air: *pulsatilla 30*, Regime A1.

Glue ear perhaps with some loss of hearing; discharge perhaps offensive; patient irritable, chilly and sensitive to cold: *hepar sulph 30*, Regime A1.

Ears remain blocked after a cold or ear infection: *silica 200*, Regime A2.

Constitutional treatment

A tendency to recurrent earaches, infections or blockages requires constitutional treatment, to which it generally responds well. *Calc carb*, *pulsatilla* and *sulphur* children are prone to ear problems, and so are *aurum* and *psorinum* adults. Consider them in the remedy section and see the constitutional remedy finder for more suggestions. If a remedy is clearly indicated: that remedy potency 200, Regime C between attacks. Otherwise, consult a homoeopath.

ECZEMA

Specific remedies for eczema

First signs of eczema in plump, placid children: *calc carb 30*, Regime A2.

First signs of eczema in warm, boisterous children: *sulphur 30*, Regime A2.

First signs of eczema in clingy children: *pulsatilla 30*, Regime A2.

Eczema where the skin splits with a light brown discharge: *graphities 30*, Regime A.

Eczema where the skin cracks and becomes very sore, particularly in winter: *petroleum 30*, Regime A.

Eczema after grief: *ignatia 200*, Regime A2.

If nothing else has worked or is indicated and there is a delay before constitutional treatment can begin, as a means of giving some relief in the meantime: *morgan co 30*, Regime A2.

Local applications for eczema

As an antiseptic and to promote healing: *calendula cream*, Regime M, or *mother tincture*, Regime N.

To relieve the itching of eczema: *stellaria cream*, Regime M.

Constitutional treatment

In general eczema requires constitutional treatment, taking into account the physiological and psychological features of the individual. See the constitutional remedy finder for suggestions. If a remedy is clearly indicated: that remedy potency 30, Regime B during attacks, or potency 200, Regime C, between them. In general, it is highly advisable to consult a homoeopath.

This is particularly true if conventional medication is being used, especially steroid creams, or if the eczema is associated with other problems such as asthma. In such cases homoeopathic remedies can bring relief and reduce the reliance on medication, but this requires sustained and careful treatment.

EXHAUSTION, FATIGUE, WEAKNESS
(Also see Memory Loss; Chronic Fatigue)

After a period of intense physical exertion: *arnica 30*, Regime A1.

After a period of intense mental exertion, nervous exhaustion; small tasks seem overwhelming; desire to be alone and not make conversation: *kali phos 30*, Regime A1.

After a period of intense mental exhaustion, nervous exhaustion; irritable and fastidious about little things; strong desire for coffee or other stimulants: *nux vomica 30*, Regime A1.

After a period of intense emotions, left feeling drained, numb, apathetic: *phosphoric acid 30*, Regime A1.

After an acute illness, especially if a lot of fluid was lost: *china 30*, Regime A1.

After an acute illness, left feeling weak, sleepy, unsteady, perhaps aching in the back or limbs: *gelsemium 30*, Regime A1.

After a binge or sustained period of overindulgence, feeling oversensitive, irritable, perhaps with delirium tremens: *nux vomica 30*, Regime A1.

After a binge or sustained period of overindulgence, feeling sluggish, bloated: *carbo veg 30*, Regime A1.

From nursing children or after a long period of looking after someone sick and in need of constant care and attention: *cocculus 30*, Regime A1.

Exhaustion or disorientation from lack of sleep for any reason: *cocculus 30*, Regime A1.

Individualised and constitutional treatment

Apart from the remedies mentioned above there are a great number that could be indicated according to the situation and condition of the patient. So if none of these are appropriate or effective, do consult a homoeopath. Effective treatment can ensure that the period of weakness and recovery is not too long, and that it does not develop into one of the forms of chronic fatigue.

EYE INJURIES

Severe blow or injury to the eye; it is not yet clear what damage has been done: *arnica 200*, Regime G.

Black eyes from blows to the face: *arnica 30*, Regime H.

Black eyes, particularly bad or slow to heal: *ledum 30*, Regime H (may be taken alongside *arnica*).

Pain or problems following a blow directly to the eyeball: *symphytum 30*, Regime A.

Pain or problems with the eyes following a shock or exposure to very bright light: *aconite 200*, Regime A2.

Burst blood vessel causing much redness to the white of the eye; to promote healing and reabsorption: *hamamelis 30*, Regime H.

EYE PROBLEMS
(Also see Eye Infections)

Cataracts
The simplest and apparently most effective treatment for this condition is: *cineraria mother tincture*, Regime J. This seems to help in many cases if kept up for a few months.

If this does not help much, the following was recommended by Dr John Clarke: one dose of *silica 200*, followed one week later by one dose of *calc fluor 200*, followed one week later by one dose of *sulphur 200*, and then start again at the beginning. Review after three months.

Eye strain
Sore eyes, perhaps with some blurring of vision, after a period of long close work with the eyes, perhaps in poor light: *ruta 30*, Regime A.

Glaucoma
During the first symptoms or an acute flare-up of glaucoma, eyes feeling hot and sore, sensitive to light: *belladonna 30*, Regime D.

Long-standing glaucoma in lightly-built, sociable individuals: *phosphorus 30*, Regime F.

And see the note on constitutional treatment below.

Watering eyes
(Also see Eyes, Infections and Allergies; Colds)

Eyes very watery, no pain or signs of infection: *euphrasia 30*, Regime A.

Watery eyes when in the open air, in people who otherwise like a lot of fresh air: *pulsatilla 30*, Regime A.

And see the note on constitutional treatment below.

Dry eyes

During a cold or other infectious, short-term condition: *belladonna 30*, Regime A1.

In sad, sensitive individuals: *natrum mur 200*, Regime C.

And see the note on constitutional treatment below.

Loss of vision

After injury to the eye: *arnica 200*, Regime A3.

After shock or fright: *aconite 200*, Regime A3.

After grief: *ignatia 200*, Regime A3.

Gradual blurring of vision from impaired blood supply to the eye: *hamamelis 30*, Regime F.

Constitutional treatment

Long-standing cases of any of the above conditions may respond to constitutional treatment. See the constitutional remedy finder for suggestions. If a remedy is clearly indicated: that remedy potency 30, Regime A. In most cases treatment would have to be precise and kept up for a long period in order to make a real difference, so do consult a homoeopath.

EYES, INFECTIONS AND ALLERGIC REACTIONS
(Also see Allergies)

Eye infections, conjunctivitis (may be part of a cold or other condition)

Simple infection or inflammation of the eye, with redness and profuse clear discharge; eyes may be itching or burning: *euphrasia 30*, Regime A1.

Eye infection or conjunctivitis, with a thick white, yellow or green discharge; the patient is in a placid or weepy state of mind: *pulsatilla 30*, Regime A1.

Eye infection with a thin, runny, green or foul-looking discharge; patient perhaps in a bad-tempered, unpredictable mood; maybe hot or clammy sweats: *mercurius 30*, Regime A1.

Eye infection with a thin, runny, green or foul-looking discharge; patient hot, perhaps in a restless, anxious state of mind: *argent nit 30*, Regime A1.

If any of the above do not help or only slightly or temporarily, they
may be usefully followed by: *medorrhinum 200*, Regime C.
And see the note on constitutional treatment below.

Allergic reactions
Sudden allergic reaction involving the eyes; great swelling around the
eye, as if the area were full of fluid; hot, red and shiny; cool air or
applications relieve the discomfort, particularly if the upper lid is most
affected: *apis 200*, Regime D.
Sudden allergic reaction of the eyes, with great swelling around the
eye; if warm applications are soothing or if the lower lid is clearly more
affected than the upper: *arsen alb 200*, Regime D.

Constitutional treatment

Long-standing or repeated episodes of these conditions require constitutional treatment, to which they often respond well. See the constitutional remedy finder for suggestions. If a remedy is clearly indicated:
that remedy potency 30, Regime B during attacks, or potency 200,
Regime C between them. Otherwise consult a homoeopath.

FEAR AND ANXIETY
(Also see Shock and Fright; Confidence Lacking)

Panic attacks: *aconite 200*, Regime B2.
A big event is coming up, feeling unusually lacking in confidence,
paralysed by nerves: *gelsemium 30*, Regime B1.
A big event is coming up, or fear of specific things such as flying,
feeling really terrified about the ordeal ahead: *aconite 200*, Regime
B1.
A big event is coming up, or that kind of feeling for no apparent reason;
feeling hot, restless; irrational thoughts of the 'what if' kind keep
invading the mind; perhaps comfort eating: *argent nit 30*, Regime
B1.
Nightmares or frightening images keep coming into the mind after a
horrible experience (even horror films); violent thoughts, fear of the
dark and being alone: *stramonium 200*, Regime B.
Nightmares or fears after a horrible experience, mixed with jealousy or
sexuality; violent thoughts, fear of losing control: *hyoscyamus 200*,
Regime C.

Recurring attacks of anxiety in conscientious individuals: *arsen alb 200*, Regime C.

Recurring attacks of anxiety behind a haughty or stern exterior, causing gastric disturbances with much flatulence; worse before important events: *lycopodium 200*, Regime C.

Panic attacks during the menopause: *aconite 200*, Regime B2.

Constitutional treatment

If none of the above are appropriate or effective, or if the relief is only temporary, constitutional treatment is needed. Any constitutional type may be afflicted by anxiety; among those most prone are *argent nit*, *arsen alb*, *calc carb*, *hyoscyamus*, *lycopodium*, *phosphorus*, *psorinum*, *silica* and *stramonium*. Consider them in the remedy section, and see the constitutional remedy finder for more suggestions. If a remedy is clearly indicated: that remedy potency 200, Regime C. Careful homoeopathic treatment over a sustained period can make a big difference, but as it is difficult to be objective about one's own anxieties it is very worthwhile consulting a homoeopath.

FEMALE REPRODUCTIVE SYSTEM PROBLEMS
(Also see Fibroids; Period Problems; Sexual Problems; Vaginal Conditions)

Constitutional and individualised treatment

Endometriosis, fibroids, ovarian cysts, tumours and other conditions of the female sexual organs often respond well to constitutional treatment. *Apis*, *kali carb*, *lachesis*, *lilium tig*, *phosphorus*, *pulsatilla*, and *sepia* types are among those most prone to such conditions. Consider them in the remedy section and see the constitutional remedy finder for suggestions. If a remedy is clearly indicated: that remedy potency 30, Regime A. Otherwise consult a homoeopath. In general, this is highly advisable.

FEVER, HIGH TEMPERATURE, PYREXIA

This section covers just the stage where high temperature is the major symptom. If a cough, cold, flu, childhood disease or any other condition should develop, see the appropriate section.

High fevers

Fever with fits, delirium, severe pain or a temperature of 40°C (104°F) or over: *aconite 200*, Regime G.

Fever with a temperature of 39°C (102°F) or over, skin bright red and hot to touch, pupils dilated, dizziness: *belladonna 200*, Regime D.

Fever with a temperature of 39°C (102°F) or over, skin hot and dry, restless, anxious state of mind, thirsty: *aconite 200*, Regime D.

Moderate fevers

Child or adult has a fever which came on suddenly in the last few hours; skin hot and dry; restless, anxious state of mind; thirsty, perhaps dry cough: *aconite 30*, Regime B2.

Child or adult has a fever which came on quickly in the last 48 hours; skin dry and hot to touch, pupils dilated, dizziness, better sitting up: *belladonna 30*, Regime B3.

Child has a fever which came on suddenly in the last few hours; skin hot and dry; very bad temper, the child demands to be carried and comforted continuously; perhaps teething, perhaps with diarrhoea: *chamomilla 30*, Regime B3.

Child or adult has a fever which came on gradually in the last 48 hours; perhaps started with sore throat; feeling tired and apathetic, few clear symptoms: *ferrum phos 30*, Regime B1.

Fever with nausea; weak and tired; thirsty but drinks only a little at a time; restless and anxious state of mind, does not want to be left alone; chilly and wants warmth (except perhaps to the head): *arsen alb 30*, Regime B1.

Fever; pains in head or chest made worse by moving; irritable, just want to be at home and quiet; thirsty for long drinks: *bryonia 30*, Regime B1.

Fever; aching or heaviness in the limbs or back; drowsy and listless; not thirsty, perhaps sore throat: *gelsemium 30*, Regime B1.

Homoeopathy and fevers

Whenever there is a problem in the body the two most common symptoms are inflammation of the affected part, if there is one, and general fever in the system as a whole. Both are effects of the body reacting to the problem, as well as signs that something is wrong. Fever is almost always a symptom of an acute (short-term, self-limiting) disease, rather than of chronic (long-term) conditions, although acute flare-ups of chronic conditions may involve fever.

Modern drugs are effective at turning off the mechanisms that produce fever, and thus reducing body temperature. This does lessen the possibility of convulsions and other complications, but clearly it does not address the underlying cause and is an interference in the body's natural self-defences, which are what homoeopathy tries (and sometimes fails) to augment and support. Exactly how and when it is best to intervene in fevers is one of many fundamental medical issues where there are as yet no clear scientific formulas to guide us.

FIBROIDS, UTERINE

Specific remedy
Fraxinus americana mother tincture, Regime E2.

Constitutional treatment

Constitutional treatment should be pursued with, or in preference to, the above remedy. See the section on female reproductive organ problems.

FISSURES, ANAL

Fissure or tears of the anus from large or hard stools, to help the area to heal as quickly as possible: *hamamelis 30*, Regime H. (May be given alongside individualised treatment as outlined below.)
Anal fissure after emotional upset or during infectious illness; intense pain on passing stool: *nitric acid 30*, Regime A.

Local application
As well as the above, *calendula cream*, Regime M.

Individualised and constitutional treatment

If the suggestions above are not appropriate or effective, constitutional treatment is needed. *Graphities*, *nitric acid*, *silica* and *thuja* types are among those prone to fissures. Consider them in the remedy section, and see the constitutional remedy finder for suggestions. If a remedy is clearly indicated: that remedy potency 30, Regime A during episodes, or potency 200, Regime C in between. Otherwise see a homoeopath.

FITS, CONVULSIONS, EPILEPSY

Child with a high temperature goes into a fit, is very red, hot to the touch, delirious, pupils dilated: *belladonna 200*, Regime G (give after or between convulsions).

Child with high temperature goes into a fit, violent movements, fists clenched, skin goes blue: *cuprum met 200*, Regime G (give after or between convulsions).

An adult goes into a fit without warning: *cuprum met 200*, Regime G (give after or between convulsions).

An adult feels the symptoms of a fit coming on, warns those around what to expect: *cicuta 200*, Regime I.

Regular fits in individuals with severe learning difficulties and/or sexual precocity: *bufo 30*, Regime G on the onset of fits, *bufo 200*, Regime C in between.

Fits from fright: *aconite 200*, Regime D.

Fits from emotional distress: *ignatia 200*, Regime D.

Constitutional treatment

The tendency to have regular fits or epilepsy needs constitutional treatment between episodes, if at all possible before anticonvulsion drugs are started, although treatment is not impossible later. *Argent nit*, *causticum*, *cuprum* and *hyoscyamus* types are prone to this kind of problem. Consider them in the remedy section, and see the constitutional remedy finder for more suggestions. If a remedy is clearly indicated: that remedy potency 200, Regime C between attacks. In general, it is advisable to consult a homoeopath.

FLATULENCE, ABDOMINAL BLOATING
(Also see Abdominal Pain; Bowels and Colon Problems)

Remedies for short-term relief

Flatulence, bloating, after a big meal or overindulgence, feeling heavy and sluggish: *carbo veg 30*, Regime B1.

Flatulence, bloating, after a big meal or overindulgence; perhaps desire to pass wind or burp but unable to do so completely; irritable: *nux vomica 30*, Regime B1.

Tendency to flatulence and bloating; craving for sweet things which make the problem worse; hot, agitated, restless state of mind: *argent nit 30*, Regime B1.

Tendency to flatulence and bloating; craving for sweet things which make the problem worse; feeling anxious as if a big event is coming up; symptoms particularly bad in the late afternoon; discomfort in the abdomen worse on the right side: *lycopodium 30*, Regime B1.

Tendency to flatulence and bloating; most of the gas is trapped; feeling exhausted; in fastidious, anxious, sensitive individuals even if they are careful about diet: *china 30*, Regime B1.

Flatulence or bloating after any meal, however carefully one eats, gas may be trapped; perhaps feeling lethargic; or none of the above remedies are indicated: *carbo veg 30*, Regime B1.

Constipation with flatulence or bloating, strong urge to pass stool but only gas is produced: *carbo veg 30*, Regime B1.

Constitutional treatment

Recurrent or stubborn bouts of flatulence generally respond well to constitutional treatment. *Argent nit*, *carbo veg*, *china*, and *lycopodium* are the types most prone of all to this problem. Consider them in the remedy section and see the constitutional remedy finder for more suggestions. If a remedy is clearly indicated: that remedy potency 30, Regime B1 during attacks, or potency 200, Regime C between them. Otherwise consult a homoeopath.

FLUID RETENTION, OEDEMA
(Also see Kidney Problems)

Fluid retention during illness, hot weather, or for no apparent reason, patient not thirsty and intolerant of heat: *apis 30*, Regime B1.

Fluid retention during illness, patient is thirsty and cold, urinating very little: *apocynam can 30*, Regime B1.

Swelling of the hands, feet or perhaps limbs, where the patient is rather debilitated and chilly: *kali carb 30*, Regime A.

Fluid retention in pregnancy or during periods, generally better in fresh air; tearful or placid mood: *pulsatilla 30*, Regime A1.

Fluid retention in pregnancy or during periods, generally chilly and better for warmth; irritable, unsociable mood: *sepia 30*, Regime A1.

Fluid retention while flying: *coca 30*, Regime A1.

Generalised fluid retention with long-term kidney problems: *natrum mur 30*, Regime A.

Constitutional treatment

A tendency to fluid retention requires constitutional treatment. *Apis, arsen alb, china, lycopodium, kali carb, natrum mur* and *sepia* types are among those most prone to the problem. Consider them in the remedy section, and see the constitutional remedy finder for suggestions. If a remedy is clearly indicated: that remedy potency 30, Regime A. Otherwise consult a homoeopath.

FUNGAL INFECTIONS, SKIN
(Also see Dermatitis)

Athlete's foot, fungal infection of the groin, or similar skin problem; or fungal infection around the nails: *silica 30*, Regime F2.
Short-term skin eruption diagnosed as fungal, in slightly-built, dry-skinned individuals: *silica 30*, Regime A.
Short-term skin eruption diagnosed as fungal, in other types: *sulphur 30*, Regime A.

Local applications
If the skin is broken: *hypericum and calendula mother tincture*, Regime N1, alongside any of the above.
If the skin is not broken: *propolis mother tincture*, Regime N1, alongside any of the above.

Individualised and constitutional treatment

Fungal infections cover a wide range of skin problems which are thought not to be either bacteriological or viral. Homoeopathic treatment is mostly constitutional, according to the nature of the eruption and mostly on the circumstances and nature of the person with it. *Calc carb, silica, staphisagria, sulphur* and *thuja* types are among those particularly prone to this kind of skin condition. Consider them in the remedy section, and see the constitutional remedy finder for suggestions. If a remedy is clearly indicated: that remedy potency 30, Regime A. Otherwise see a homoeopath.

GALL BLADDER PROBLEMS

Tendency to form gallstones, threatening to cause colic or require surgery
In slightly-built individuals: *silica 30*, Regime F1.
In heavily-built individuals: *calc carb 30*, Regime F1.

Gallstone colic
Pains around the area of the liver, extending backwards or to between the shoulder-blades: *chelidonium 30*, Regime B3.
Sharp, cutting pains radiating around area of liver, worse for movement or pressure: *berberis 30*, Regime B3.

Constitutional treatment

For recurrent attacks of gallstone colic, or if the gall bladder is not working well and insufficient bile is causing digestive troubles, constitutional treatment might help. *China, lycopodium, natrum sulph* and *nux vomica* types are among those most prone to gall bladder problems. See them in the remedy section and the constitutional remedy finder for suggestions. If a remedy is well indicated: that remedy potency 30, Regime F1. Otherwise consult a homoeopath.

GERMAN MEASLES (RUBELLA)

Early stages
In the early stages, before the glands have swollen or rash appeared and diagnosis is confirmed: see Fever.

Later stages
Patient placid, weepy and wanting attention. Warm and not very thirsty: *pulsatilla 30*, Regime L.
The patient is quite lively when given lots of attention, very unhappy if left alone; thirsty: *phosphorus 30*, Regime L.
Swollen glands behind the ears are particularly painful, or there is pain in the throat extending to the ears on swallowing: *phytolacca 30*, Regime L.

Prevention

If a child has been in contact with someone with German Measles, most homoeopaths believe that the best thing is to allow the immune response to proceed naturally. However, if for some reason it is wished to do all possible to prevent it occurring at this time: *rubella 30*, Regime K (see *nosodes,* p. 197).

If a woman in the first three months of pregnancy, has not had the disease or been immunised and is in any danger of coming into contact with it and wishes to use homoeopathic *nosodes* (see *nosodes,* p. 197) alongside appropriate medical treatment: *rubella 30,* Regime K. If in contact, repeat while seeking advice.

GLANDULAR FEVER, MONONUCLEOSIS
(Also see Fever; Exhaustion)

Specific remedies
Glands very swollen, hard and sore, pains in throat better for cold drinks and worse for hot ones, although as a whole the patient is chilly and worse for cold; prostration, general soreness of whole body: *phytolacca 30*, Regime A.
Tired and sleepy, limbs and eyes feel heavy, aching in the limbs and back, sore throat, shaky or shivering, thirstless, perhaps came on after some bad news or with a big event coming up: *gelsemium 30*, Regime A.
Sore throat, swallowing anything is painful, nothing seems to make it better; shivering one minute, sweating the next, very sensitive to heat and cold; bad-tempered and easily offended; salivating more than usual, bad breath: *mercurius 30*, Regime A.
Glandular fever with swollen glands and sore throat, mostly severe tiredness, mentally dull and confused, symptoms rather like the generalised infection of influenza or food poisoning but symptoms do not change or develop over time: *ailanthus gland 30*, Regime A.
Glandular fever where there are few clear symptoms apart from perhaps some swelling of the glands and mostly just great prostration: *carcinosin 200*, Regime C.
Old cases that have lasted weeks or months with few symptoms apart from extreme tiredness, particularly in individuals with a previous history of emotional strain or prolonged mental exertion: *carcinosin 200*, Regime C.

Individualised and constitutional treatment

Severe or recurrent cases that do not respond to any of the suggestions above need individualised and probably constitutional treatment to take into account the physiological and psychological factors that are draining the individual's energy. See the constitutional remedy finder for suggestions. If a remedy is clearly indicated: that remedy potency 200, Regime C. This condition usually responds very well to accurate prescribing so in general it is advisable to consult a homoeopath.

GOUT

Occasional bouts of classic gout, severe pain in the big toe, worse for pressure or movement, and cold; perhaps when weather changes from warm to cool; perhaps high uric acid levels confirmed: *colchicum 30*, Regime A.

Gout, with dark brown, very smelly urine: *benzoic acid 30*, Regime A.

Gout come on suddenly after a binge or period of overindulgence; chilly; perhaps irritable, oversensitive state of mind: *nux vomica 30*, Regime A.

Occasional bouts of gout, none of the above indicated or effective: *urtica urens 30*, Regime A.

Acute or repeated attacks of gout in individuals with a tendency to liver or stomach problems, with much flatulence; symptoms generally worse on the right side of the body and in the late afternoon; anxiety as before a big event but for no obvious reason: *lycopodium 30*, Regime A during attacks, or *lycopodium 200*, Regime C between them.

Constitutional treatment

Long-term tendencies to repeated attacks of gout usually respond well to constitutional treatment. Apart from *lycopodium* above, see the constitutional remedy finder for suggestions. If a remedy is clearly indicated: that remedy potency 30, Regime A during attacks, or potency 200, Regime C between them. Otherwise consult a homoeopath.

GRIEF, LOSS, BEREAVEMENT, DISAPPOINTMENT
(Also see Depression)

The immediate effects of grief, loss or disappointment; pain and distress, mental disorientation, difficulty coping with things or controlling one's feelings, perhaps cannot accept it or cannot believe it, perhaps unable to cry: *ignatia 200*, Regime A.

The effects of grief about something that happened six weeks ago or more, grieving incomplete or unresolved, cannot or will not weep, desire to be alone or only with those who really understand and sympathise; self-reproach, irritable about trivia: *natrum mur 200*, Regime C.

The effects of grief about something that happened six weeks ago or more, now feeling only numb, apathetic and indifferent to everything; physical and mental exhaustion after grief or distress: *phosphoric acid 30*, Regime A.

The effects of grief or loss for something that happened six weeks ago or more, complete and deep depression, feeling that death would almost be a relief and only the sense of one's duties keeps one going; melancholic introspection: *aurum met 200*, Regime C.

The immediate or long-term effects of grief, loss or disappointment when the feelings are very much mixed up with anger, outrage or violation, particularly if it cannot be acted upon and the anger and sense of injustice inhibit the grieving process: *staphisagria 200*, Regime C.

Individualised and constitutional treatment

Sometimes the effect of mental trauma is to bring out symptoms of the individual's constitutional type, in which case it is constitutional treatment that is needed. See the constitutional remedy finder for suggestions. If a remedy is clearly indicated: that remedy potency 200, Regime C. Otherwise see a homoeopath. In general conditions of this kind respond well to homoeopathic treatment, but remedies have to be accurately prescribed so it is advisable to consult a homoeopath.

GUM DISEASE

Remedies for occasional sore gums
Occasional episodes of gums becoming acutely sore, ulcerated or

inflamed, bleeding easily, perhaps bad breath, tongue flabby and indented: *mercurius 30*, Regime A.

Occasional episodes of gums becoming sore and bleeding easily, perhaps infected, painful if touched, pain worse for cold things, better for warmth: *hepar sulph 30*, Regime A.

Recurrent or persistent gum problems

Gums generally tending to recede or become inflamed; in slightly-built, dry-skinned, chilly, mild-tempered individuals: *silica 30*, Regime F1.

Gums generally tending to recede and bleed easily, in individuals with generally poor circulation; perhaps some bluish discoloration of the area: *carbo veg 30*, Regime F1.

Gums generally tending to recede or become inflamed, with a tendency to mouth ulcers, bad breath; in individuals with the sort of body type that is very sensitive to both heat and cold: *mercurius 30*, Regime F1.

Gums generally tending to recede or become inflamed, in individuals tired or strained by work, particularly mental exertion, perhaps with yellow tongue: *kali phos 30*, Regime F1.

Local application

Alongside any of the above: *calendula mother tincture*, Regime N5.

Individualised and constitutional treatment

If none of the above are appropriate or effective constitutional treatment might help, alongside the necessary dental attention. *Antim crud, calc carb, graphities, kali carb, phosphorus* and *staphisagria* types are among those prone to the problem. Consider them in the remedy section, and see the constitutional remedy finder for suggestions. If a remedy is clearly indicated: that remedy potency 30, Regime F1. Otherwise a homoeopath might be consulted. Remedies would have to be prescribed accurately and over a period of weeks or months to make a real difference.

HAEMORRHOIDS: see Piles, p. 93.

HAIR PROBLEMS: LOSS, WEAKNESS, ALOPECIA

Loss of hair after a debilitating illness, or after grief or emotional distress: *phosphoric acid 12*, Regime F1.

Loss or thinning of hair after childbirth or at the menopause: *sepia 12*,
Regime F1.
Alopecia or general loss or thinning of previously healthy hair, particu-
larly in lightly-built, dry-skinned individuals: *silica 12*, Regime F1.
Alopecia or general loss or thinning of previously healthy hair, particu-
larly in fully-built, soft-skinned individuals: *calc carb 12*, Regime
F1.

Local application
Alongside any of the above: *arnica mother tincture*, Regime N3.

Constitutional treatment

If none of the suggestions above are appropriate or effective, cases of
abrupt hair loss, thinning or alopecia may respond to constitutional
treatment. See the constitutional remedy finder for suggestions and if
a remedy is clearly indicated: that remedy potency 12, Regime F1.
Otherwise consult a homoeopath. Cases of general, gradual hair loss in
men where baldness runs in the family rarely respond much to anything.

HEAD INJURIES

Immediately after the injury: *arnica 200*, Regime G or A1.
If symptoms, particularly headaches or vertigo, persist long after the
injury: *natrum sulph 200*, Regime C.

Individualised treatment

If neither of the above is effective or appropriate, consult a homoeopath
for individualised treatment.

HEADACHES, MIGRAINE

Headaches after a binge or overindulgence; hangover; sensitive to every
noise and cold; irritable mood: *nux vomica 30*, Regime B2.
Headaches or migraines where the pain is aggravated by any motion
and better if one can keep completely still; better lying alone in a
dark, quiet room; irritable; perhaps feeling hot and better for cool
air: *bryonia 200*, Regime B3.
Thumping, throbbing headache; worse in the forehead or temples; come

on suddenly; perhaps with dizziness; brought on by getting cold or by heat or the sun; pain worse for any sudden movement; perhaps worse on the right side and around 3 a.m. or 3 p.m.: *belladonna 30*, Regime B3.

Headaches or migraines with or preceded by disturbance or loss of vision and/or nausea; tend to recur at fairly regular intervals such as weekly; head feels hot and full; pain worse when lying down; better moving around gently; perhaps worse on the right side: *iris ves 30*, Regime B3.

Recurrent headaches in sensitive, reserved individuals; perhaps beginning or centred in the neck; everything feels dry and tense; perhaps brought on after unexpressed emotions; strong wish to be alone or with someone who understands: *natrum mur 200*, Regime B3.

Headaches from studying or intense mental work: *nux vomica 30*, Regime B.

Headaches after a blow or injury to the head: *natrum sulph 200*, Regime A2.

Headaches during periods: see Period Problems, p. 91, and consider particularly *sepia*, *natrum mur* and *belladonna* in the remedy section. If one is clearly appropriate: potency 30, Regime B.

Headaches during the menopause: consider *belladonna*, *lachesis*, *natrum mur* and *sepia* in the remedy section. If one is clearly appropriate: potency 30, Regime B.

Headaches with anger: see Anger, p. 21, and consider particularly *staphisagria* and *colocynth* in the remedy section. If one is clearly appropriate: potency 30, Regime B.

Constitutional treatment

Recurrent headaches require constitutional treatment. Perhaps *lachesis*, *natrum mur*, *silica* and *sulphur* are the greatest headache remedies, but any constitutional type could suffer them. Consider the above in the remedy section and see the constitutional remedy finder for more suggestions. If a remedy is clearly indicated: that remedy potency 30, Regime B1 during attacks, or potency 200, Regime C between them. The tendency to suffer headaches and migraines usually responds very well to careful homoeopathic treatment so consulting a homoeopath is worthwhile and advisable.

HEARING LOST, DEAFNESS

During a cold or from blockage by wax or catarrh: see Ear Problems, p. 49.
Hearing reduced after a shock or bad news: *gelsemium 200*, Regime C.
Hearing reduced after exposure to loud noise: *hypericum 1M*, Regime K, followed by *kali phos 30*, Regime F2.

Constitutional treatment

For gradual loss of hearing with advancing age there is little that homoeopathy can do. In cases of early or abrupt hearing loss, constitutional treatment might help. See the constitutional remedy finder for suggestions. If a remedy is clearly indicated: that remedy potency 200, Regime C. Otherwise consult a homoeopath. In order to make a real difference remedies would have to be prescribed very accurately.

HEART ATTACK, MYOCARDIAL INFARCTION
(Also see Heart Conditions)

Suspected heart attack, classic symptoms of heart attack, severe pain in the chest extending to both shoulders and particularly down the left arm, perhaps numbness and coldness of the fingers: *latrodectus mac 200*, Regime G.
Severe pains as if the heart were being squeezed in wires, heaviness of the chest and breathlessness, anxiety, pain perhaps extending to left arm, worse lying on the left side: *cactus grand 200*, Regime G.
Suspected heart attack, oppression of chest, breathlessness, severe anxiety: *arsen alb 200*, Regime G.
Person has had a heart attack, now recovering; to promote recovery and minimise short-term danger of recurrences: *arnica 6* and *kali mur 6*, Regime H1.

Constitutional treatment

If there is a history of heart attacks it is highly advisable to seek constitutional treatment to optimise health and minimise the danger of recurrences.

HEART CONDITIONS
(Also see Heart Attack; Blood Pressure, High and Low)

Pains in the region of the heart, angina
Classic symptoms of angina or heart attack; severe pain in the chest
   extending to both shoulders and particularly down the left arm; perhaps numbness and coldness of the fingers: *latrodectus mac 200*,
   Regime G if suspected heart attack; potency 30, Regime B1
   otherwise.
Severe pains as if the heart were being squeezed in wires; heaviness of
   the chest and breathlessness; anxiety; pain perhaps extending to left
   arm, worse lying on the left side: *cactus grand 30*, Regime B1.
Pains around the heart; with slow pulse; pains and feeling that the heart
   might stop beating; symptoms worse for any exertion or excitement;
   perhaps diagnosed congestive heart disease; pains perhaps extending
   to left arm: *digitalis 30*, Regime B1.
Pains around the heart with powerful palpitations; pain on the left side
   and worse lying on the left; desire for hot drinks: *spigelia 30*, Regime
   B1.
Pains around the heart; worse on the right side and going into the right
   arm; palpitations felt in chest or any part of the body; in hot, busy,
   discontented individuals: *lilium tig 30*, Regime B1.
Also see constitutional treatment, p. 71.

Palpitations
Palpitations after a binge or sustained overindulgence of stimulants
   including coffee; feeling irritable, oversensitive: *nux vomica 30*,
   Regime B1.
Palpitations from fright or shock: *aconite 200*, Regime B2.
Palpitations from grief or distress: *ignatia 200*, Regime B2.
Palpitations from happy news or overexcitement: *coffea 200*, Regime
   B2.
Palpitations that come on or last for an oddly long time after physical
   exertion: *lycopus 30*, Regime B2.
Palpitations in the sun: *belladonna 30*, Regime B2.
Violent palpitations or pulsations felt in any part of the body; pains
   around the heart; worse on the right side and going into the right arm;
   in hot, dissatisfied individuals, particularly with hormonal imbalance:
   lilium tig 30, Regime B1.

Palpitations during the menopause: consider in particular *lachesis, lilium tig* and *glonoine* as described in the remedy section. If one is clearly appropriate: potency 30, Regime B1.

Also see constitutional treatment, below.

Irregular heart rate; arrhythmias

Occasional racing heart from fear or with great anxiety: *aconite 200*, Regime D.

Where the pulse is irregular, intermittent and generally slow, perhaps other symptoms of heart disease like weakness and cold extremities; perhaps with metabolic problems as well as the slow pulse; anxiety, fear of the heart stopping: *digitalis 30*, Regime B1.

Pulse irregular and rather weak; perhaps some pain under the left shoulder blade or left collar bone. As a general tonic to the heart where there are signs of strain or weakness, or if thickening of the arteries is suspected: *crateagus mother tincture*, Regime E1.

Violent palpitations with pain in the heart like being squeezed: *cactus grand 30*, Regime B3.

Palpitations with anxiety; need to breath deeply; perhaps after habitual use of much alcohol or caffeine; worse in the dark; symptoms worse from exertion and strong emotions: *strophanthus 30*, Regime B3.

Also see constitutional treatment below.

Thickening of the arteries; arteriosclerosis

Heart conditions or poor circulation with suspected thickening of the arteries: *crateagus mother tincture*, Regime E1.

Constitutional treatment of heart conditions

Apart from the suggestions above, it is constitutional treatment that is most likely to relieve these conditions when they occur, as well as the tendency to get them. Often such symptoms are the first sign that something is wrong before any physical damage sets in and it is at this stage that constitutional treatment is most effective in resolving problems and avoiding more serious conditions developing in future.

Among the constitutional types that are most prone to heart conditions are *apis, arsen alb, argent nit, aurum met, lachesis, lilium tig, natrum mur, pulsatilla* and *sulphur* types. Consider them in the remedy section, and see the constitutional remedy finder for more suggestions. If a remedy is clearly indicated: that remedy potency 30, Regime B2 during attacks, or potency 200, Regime C between them. In general it is worthwhile and recommended that you consult a homoeopath.

HERPES, GENITAL

Occasional outbreaks of genital herpes, made worse when tired or vexed, and by sexual activity: *natrum mur 200*, Regime K between episodes.

Occasional outbreaks of genital herpes, when there seems to be no discernible pattern to the occurrences: *thuja 200*, Regime K between episodes.

During outbreaks, to minimise the duration and discomfort, where the eruptions are dry and cracked: *petroleum 30*, Regime A.

During outbreaks, to minimise the duration and discomfort, where the eruptions are moist, red bumps: *rhus tox 30*, Regime A.

Constitutional and individualised treatment

If none of the above are appropriate or effective, constitutional treatment might help. Consider the *calc carb*, *graphities*, *mercurius*, *natrum mur*, *sepia* and *thuja* types as described in the remedy section of this book. If one is clearly indicated: that remedy potency 30, Regime A during attacks or potency 200, Regime C between them. Remedies have to be prescribed accurately over a sustained period to make a real difference to this condition.

HICCOUGHS

Hiccoughs after eating too much or too quickly: *nux vomica 30*, Regime B1.

After intense emotions: *ignatia 30*, Regime B1.

Constitutional treatment

Prolonged or recurrent bouts of troublesome hiccoughs need constitutional treatment. See the constitutional remedy finder for suggestions. If a remedy is clearly indicated: that remedy potency 30, Regime B1 during attacks, or potency 200, Regime C between them. Otherwise see a homoeopath.

HOT FLUSHES, MENOPAUSAL

(For other problems associated with the menopause, see Fear and Anxiety; Headaches; Heart Conditions, palpitations).

With mood swings, irrational temper, depression, sudden weeping, great desire to be alone and quiet, averse to sex and physical contact; in chilly individuals: *sepia 30*, Regime A.

With mood swings, irrational temper, suspicious and jealous, strong opinions about everything and have to express them; hot, cannot bear tight clothing: *lachesis 30*, Regime A.

Moods alternate between placidity and irrational weeping, strong desire for supportive company; cannot bear stuffy places: *pulsatilla 30*, Regime A.

Irritable, introspective and miserable, strong desire to be alone, sad but unable to weep; headaches, craving for salty foods: *natrum mur 30*, Regime A.

Few mental or physical symptoms apart from the hot flushes or night sweats: *amyl nitrate 30*, Regime H2.

Few mental or physical symptoms apart from the hot flushes or night sweats; flushes cause pain or headaches: *glonoine 30*, Regime H2.

If nothing else helps: *salvia (sage) mother tincture*, Regime E5.

Potentised oestrogen

Some improvement has been reported in otherwise difficult cases by using oestrogen prepared like a homoeopathic remedy. This can be done alongside other remedies. A typical regime is: *oestrogen 6*, Regime F1.

Constitutional and individualised treatment

Treatment of hot flushes and any other problems during the menopause often needs a mixture of constitutional and specific remedies. *Apis, kali carb, lachesis, lilium tig, natrum mur, sepia* and *sulphur* are among the types most prone to these conditions. Consider them in the remedy section and see the constitutional remedy finder for suggestions. If a remedy is well indicated: that remedy potency 30, Regime A. Otherwise it is recommended that you see a homoeopath.

HYPERACTIVITY

Occasional episodes of hyperactivity such as during the seasonal festivities or after consuming too much sugary food: *coffea 200*, Regime A2.

Hyperactivity, with love of dancing or rapid movement, especially to loud and rhythmical music (such as that atavistic cacophany popular with the contemporary young), the child resists all restraints and dislikes physical contact; perhaps with twitching or pins and needles: *tarantula hisp 200*, Regime C.

Precocious children with a mean, destructive streak if they are bored; intelligent but lacking concentration; skinny despite big appetite; tendency to chest complaints or allergies, perhaps oddly frightened of cats and dogs; perhaps tooth-grinders: *tuberculinum 200*, Regime C.

Constitutional and individualised treatment

Generally hyperactivity needs constitutional treatment. Apart from *tarantula* and *tuberculinum*, among the remedies most often prescribed for this condition are *arsen iod*, *belladonna*, *hyoscyamus*, *iodum*, *medorrhinum* and *stramonium*. See them in the remedy section of this book and if one is clearly indicated: that remedy potency 200, Regime C. Otherwise see a homoeopath. Assuming any dietary and environmental factors have been addressed, homoeopathic treatment can make a significant difference in this condition, but remedies have to be prescribed accurately over a sustained period.

HYPOGLYCAEMIA, (LOW BLOOD SUGAR LEVELS)

Specific remedies

Classic symptoms of hypoglycaemia; shaking, pulse rate increased, breathless, light-headed, perhaps irritable, and craving sugary foods: *sulphur 30*, Regime B2 alongside appropriate food intake.

If attacks tend to happen during or just after times of strong emotion: *ignatia 30*, Regime B2 alongside appropriate food intake.

Constitutional treatment

The suggestions above are just measures to minimise the intensity and duration of individual attacks. The tendency for them to happen needs constitutional treatment. *Argent nit, lycopodium, natrum mur, phosphorus* and *sulphur* are among the constitutional types most potentially prone to the problem. Consider them as described in the remedy section, and see the constitutional remedy finder for more suggestions. If a remedy is clearly indicated: that remedy potency 200, Regime C. This condition often responds well to careful treatment, so in general it is advisable to consult a homoeopath.

On the treatment of metabolic conditions
The note on the homoeopathic treatment of these conditions in the section on Diabetes (p. 48) may be of interest.

IMPETIGO

Classic case of impetigo, bubbly eruptions burst leaving scabby crusts, usually around the mouth or nose; the child or patient is irritable and particularly does not want to be looked at: *antim crud 30*, Regime A.
Where the eruptions are itchy, worse for warmth and bathing; the patient is irritable and lazy: *sulphur 30*, Regime A.
The area is sore and raw, the child cannot or will not leave it alone, constantly picks at the area perhaps causing it to bleed: *arum triph 30*, Regime A.
Area cracked and oozing pus, itching, perhaps with the odd symptom that the itch moves to somewhere else if scratched, particularly if the scalp is affected: *mezereum 30*, Regime A.

Local application
Besides any of the above: *calendula mother tincture*, Regime N1 if possible, or Regime N if the former stings too much.

Constitutional and individualised treatment

A tendency to get repeated attacks of impetigo needs constitutional treatment. See the constitutional remedy finder for suggestions. If a remedy is clearly indicated: that remedy potency 200, Regime C between outbreaks. Otherwise consult a homoeopath.

INCONTINENCE
(Also see Bed-wetting)

Gradual onset of occasional incontinence on coughing, sneezing, laughing or similar stress: *causticum 30*, Regime F.

Incontinence after surgery: *staphisagria 30*, Regime F.

Incontinence during or after pregnancy, in anxious, chilly individuals: *arsen alb 30*, Regime A.

Incontinence during or after pregnancy, in placid, warm individuals: *pulsatilla 30*, Regime A.

Constitutional and individualised treatment

If none of the above are appropriate or effective, constitutional treatment could help. See the constitutional remedy finder for suggestions. If a remedy is clearly indicated: that remedy potency 30, Regime F if the condition is occasional and coming on gradually, potency 200, Regime C if it has just recently come on quite suddenly. Otherwise consult a homoeopath.

INFLUENZA

For the early stages of suspected influenza, symptoms not yet clear apart from discomfort, head cold and fever, see Colds (p. 38) and Fever (p. 56).

Aching in the limbs and back, general heaviness, eyes dull and droopy, feeling sleepy and listless; shaky and unsteady, shivery, particularly up the back; sore throat, perhaps oddly thirstless: *gelsemium 30*, Regime B.

Cases where by far the worse symptom is aching in the limbs or back, perhaps particularly bad in the shins; feeling cold, perhaps bad headache: *eupatorium perf 30*, Regime B.

Severe case, with aching in the limbs and back, feeling rather disorientated and confused; perhaps nausea or even symptoms of toxicity as of food-poisoning; bad breath, body sore causing restlessness; high temperature, thirsty: *baptisia 30*, Regime B.

Aching in the limbs and back making the patient constantly move about, so very restless; sweaty, chilly and worse for any draughts; sore throat; anxiety; everything much worse at night; perhaps cold sores: *rhus tox 30*, Regime B.

Very unstable temperature, alternately hot and cold, shivering and sweating, never comfortable; state of mind also very sensitive and changeable; sore throat, bad breath; foul temper; perhaps mouth ulcers: *mercurius 30*, Regime B.

Aching mostly in the back, with the odd symptom that in order to turn over the patient has to lean forward; chilly; irritable: *nux vomica 30*, Regime B.

Cases where one of the most troublesome symptoms is sinusitis with pain in the face and a thick, sticky nasal discharge: *kali bich 30*, Regime B.

JET-LAG

Classic symptoms of jet-lag, unpleasant feeling of disorientation, lassitude, too tired to sleep, perhaps vertigo, perhaps nausea: *cocculus 200*, Regime B.

Jet-lag, feeling as if after excessive mental or physical exertion, perhaps body aching; perhaps with strong wish just to be left alone: *arnica 200*, Regime B.

Prevention
Either of the above (or even both, in combination), Regime H6.

KIDNEY PROBLEMS
(Also see Cystitis)

Kidney stones
During attacks of kidney stone colic: *berberis 30*, Regime G during first attack, and Regime B afterwards alongside other treatment.

Tendency to form kidney stones: see constitutional treatment, p. 78.

Short-term infections and inflammations
Pain in the region of the kidneys, the pain seems to radiate into the surrounding area; worse for motion, particularly jarring movements; perhaps pain on urination: *berberis 30*, Regime B1.

Discomfort in the region of the kidneys. The feeling is fairly constant, nothing seems to change it much, no other symptoms: *berberis mother tincture*, Regime E3.

Kidney problems where swelling of limbs indicates fluid retention;

burning, sore pains when urinating; perhaps with surprisingly large quantities of urine passed, apparently more than is drunk, or hardly any is passed; the patient is not thirsty; is hot and agitated: *apis 30*, Regime B1.

The region of the kidneys remains sore and inflamed during or after a period of being unwell; urine looks smoky, and perhaps has a peculiar sweet smell, little is passed, burning pains: *terebinthina 30*, Regime B1.

Kidney troubles during acute or long-term conditions; patient craves salty things; skin dry and out of condition; tendency to headaches; patient miserable and tends to dwell on his misfortunes: *natrum mur 30*, Regime A1.

Constitutional and individualised treatment

A tendency to recurrent kidney problems often responds well to constitutional treatment besides or between any appropriate medical attention. *Apis*, *lycopodium*, *natrum mur*, *phosphorus* and *silica* types are among those most prone to such conditions. Consider them in the remedy section, and see the constitutional remedy finder for suggestions. If a remedy is clearly indicated: that remedy potency 30, Regime B1 during attacks, or potency 200, Regime C between them. In general, it is advisable to consult a homoeopath.

LEARNING DIFFICULTIES, SLOW DEVELOPMENT

These conditions sometimes respond surprisingly well to careful constitutional treatment, particularly in cases where children, for no apparent reason, just do not seem to be progressing through the usual developmental stages. By far the most important remedy in these situations is *baryta carb*. Others that can be useful include *baryta mur*, *calc phos* and *tuberculinum*. See them in the remedy section of this book, and if one is indicated: that remedy potency 200, Regime C. Otherwise consult a homoeopath.

LICE, HEAD

Local application
Staphisagria mother tincture, Regime N4.

Internal medicines
Infestations of lice are common among schoolchildren however carefully and hygienically they are cared for. Homoeopaths and parents regularly try using remedies to make individuals less susceptible to them. One often-used approach is: *bacillinum 200*, Regime F3.

LIVER PROBLEMS, HEPATITIS

Diagnosed or suspected hepatitis, discomfort in the region of the liver extending towards the back, or pain between the shoulder blades; perhaps yellow stool. If little or no jaundice is visible: *chelidonium 30*, Regime A1; if skin or eyes are clearly yellow: *chelidonium mother tincture*, Regime E3.

Diagnosed or suspected hepatitis, discomfort in the region of the liver, worse for pressure or lying on the left side; perhaps light brown or clay-coloured stool. If little or no jaundice is visible: *carduus mar 30*, Regime A1; if skin or eyes are clearly yellow: *carduus mar mother tincture*, Regime E3.

Liver disorders after a binge or period of overindulgence; patient irritable, oversensitive and chilly: *nux vomica 30*, Regime A1.

Short-term fever or disturbed digestion with liver disorder; vomiting and diarrhoea; patient anxious and restless, wanting constant company and reassurance; chilly: *asen alb 30*, Regime A1.

Apparent liver problems persisting after a bout of illness, particularly after loss of much fluid; pain in the region of the liver, worse for any touch or pressure; perhaps flatulence; patient exhausted, mentally and physically delicate: *china 30*, Regime A.

Persistent liver problems; tendency to pain in right abdomen, tendency to flatulence, symptoms worse during the late afternoon, perhaps craving for sweet foods; anxious, insecure state of mind: *lycopodium 30*, Regime A.

Persistent liver problems, tendency to diarrhoea on getting up, perhaps with headaches centred in the back of the head; the individual has a very rational approach to life but is prone to depression: *natrum sulph 30*, Regime A.

Constitutional and individualised treatment

For persistent liver troubles, constitutional treatment is needed. *Lycopodium* and *natrum sulph* are particularly prone to them; *china, mag mur, mercurius* and *phosphorus* are among the other types also predisposed to such conditions. Consider them in the remedy section, and see the constitutional remedy finder for suggestions. If a remedy is clearly indicated: that remedy potency 30, Regime A. Otherwise consult a homoeopath. These conditions generally respond well to accurate homoeopathic treatment, so it is worthwhile and advisable to see a homoeopath.

MALNUTRITION, MALABSORPTION, VITAMIN OR MINERAL DEFICIENCY

If the liver, glands, or any of the digestive organs are not working properly, see the appropriate sections.

Eating disorders may benefit from careful constitutional treatment alongside any appropriate psychotherapeutic attention.

Otherwise, a deficiency of vitamins or minerals suggests that the body is not absorbing and metabolising nutrients properly. Supplements may help in the short term, but homoeopaths usually to try to improve natural uptake from food. This requires constitutional treatment, to which such conditions often respond well. *Calc phos*, *lycopodium*, *natrum mur*, *phosphorus*, *psorinum* and *silica* are among the types most prone to poor assimilation. Consider those in the remedy section, and see the constitutional remedy finder for more suggestions. If a remedy is well indicated: that remedy potency 30 Regime F2. Treatment needs to be accurate and sustained to make a real difference, so it is advisable to see a homoeopath.

MASTITIS (INFLAMMATION OF THE BREASTS)
(Also see Breast-feeding Problems)

Condition has come on suddenly, the breast is very hot, there are red streaks radiating from the nipple, worse on the right side: *belladonna 30*, Regime B1.

In cases where any motion at all makes the pain much worse: *bryonia 30*, Regime B1.

Cases where the heat and soreness is not very intense and there is a cyst at the centre of the inflammation: *silica 30*, Regime A1.

Any cases other than those that closely fit one of the above: *phytolacca 30*, Regime B1.

During pregnancy, if none of the above are appropriate or effective, the patient is chilly and irritable: *sepia 30*, Regime A.

During pregnancy, if none of the above are appropriate or effective, the patient is hot and weepy: *pulsatilla 30*, Regime A.

Mastitis before or during the period: *phytolacca 30*, Regime B1 as above, and see note under constitutional treatment.

Constitutional treatment

Recurrent mastitis needs constitutional treatment, to which it often responds well. *Lachesis, lycopodium, mercurius, natrum mur, pulsatilla* and *sepia* types are prone to it, and *calc carb* and *tuberculinum* individuals are particularly susceptible to sore breasts just before the period. See them in the remedy section and consult the constitutional remedy finder for more suggestions. If a remedy fits well: that remedy potency 30, Regime B. Otherwise consult a homoeopath.

MEASLES

Early stages

In the early stages before eruptions have appeared and diagnosis can be confirmed: see Fever (p. 56).

Later stages

When the spots have appeared and diagnosis is confirmed, the following may be helpful.

Patient placid, weepy and wanting attention. Warm and not very thirsty: *pulsatilla 30*, Regime L. (This is very often the best remedy for the later stages of measles.)

In cases where the eyes are particularly sensitive and stream copiously: *euphrasia 30*, Regime L.

In cases where the worse symptom is a dry, painful cough: *bryonia 30*, Regime L.

The patient is quite lively when given lots of attention, very unhappy if left alone; thirsty: *phosphorus 30*, Regime L.

Prevention

If a child has been in contact with someone with measles, most homoeopaths believe that the best course is to allow the immune response to proceed naturally. However, if for some reason it is wished to do all possible to prevent it occurring at this time: *morbillinum 30*, Regime K (see *nosodes*, p. 197).

MEMORY LOSS, FORGETFULNESS, DEMENTIA, SENILITY, ALZHEIMER'S

Short-term memory loss

Short-term memory loss from overwork, strain or studying; still feeling driven to keep working, and very irritable: *nux vomica 30*, Regime A1.

Short-term memory loss from overwork, strain or studying; exhausted and highly strung, little things seem too much to cope with, jumpy: *kali phos 30*, Regime A1.

Short-term memory loss from overwork, strain or studying; body feels heavy, mind feels inert, apathy: *picric acid 30*, Regime A1.

Short-term loss or confusion of memory after a binge: *nux vomica 30*, Regime A.

Short-term loss or confusion of memory from lack of sleep: *cocculus 30*, Regime A.

Longer-term memory loss

Memory loss after an injury or blow to the head: *arnica 1M*, Regime C. If no better: *natrum sulph 1M*, Regime C.

Deterioration of memory from grief: *ignatia 200*, Regime C (and see Grief, p. 65).

Deterioration of memory after shock: *opium 200*, Regime C (and see Shock and Fright, p. 99).

Personality types prone to poor memory

Really bad memory beyond the normal limitations of ordinary human beings, which is starting to interfere with the quality of one's life, may respond to constitutional treatment. *Alumina, anacardium, argentum nit, baryta carb, lycopodium, medorrhinum* and *phosphorus* types are prone to this problem. If one of them as described in the remedy section of this book looks really appropriate: that remedy potency 200, Regime C. However, treatment has to be precise and kept up over a considerable period to make a real difference in this condition, so consulting a homoeopath is strongly recommended.

Memory loss in the elderly
Problems arise most when it is the short-term memory that is affected, leading to a breakdown of the ability to participate in life or even to care for oneself. Severe cases are labelled senility or Alzheimer's, although there are no definitive demarcations.

If the condition develops gradually from the personality types mentioned above: that remedy potency 12, Regime F1. If nothing characterises the case except a general return to the helpless state of second childhood: *baryta carb 30*, Regime F1. Otherwise, see a homoeopath. Even many experienced homoeopaths resort to the routine use of *baryta carb* for this kind of condition, partly because the personality traits that usually indicate a remedy are exactly what are breaking down.

MENOPAUSAL PROBLEMS

Advice on remedies for menopausal symptoms will be found under the following sections: Fear and Anxiety (p. 55), Headaches (p. 67), Heart Conditions—palpitations (p. 70) and Hot Flushes (p. 73). If none of the suggested remedies seem appropriate or effective, constitutional treatment is needed. *Lachesis, natrum mur, pulsatilla, sepia* and *sulphur* are some of the remedies that are most often helpful at this time. Consider them in the remedy section or consult a homoeopath.

MOLLUSCUM CONTAGIOSUM

Specific remedy
Thuja mother tincture, Regime N1, and *thuja 30*, Regime F.

Infected cases
Mollusca are a little unsightly but not usually a problem unless they get snagged on something and become infected. If this happens, see the section on abscesses and boils, and treat as such.

Constitutional treatment

Cases of molluscum are rising dramatically, and are becoming as common in children under ten as batches of warts used to be in adolescents. If *thuja* does not help, sometimes constitutional treatment will speed the rate at which they clear up—usually a few months if left untreated. *Calc carb* types seem to be prone, but this may be because so many children are *calc carb* and it is too early to judge with confidence. See the constitutional remedy finder for suggestions and if a remedy is well indicated: that remedy potency 200, Regime C. Otherwise see a homoeopath.

MUMPS

Early stages
In the early stages, before the glands have swollen and diagnosis is confirmed: see Fever, p. 56.

Later stages
High temperature, the child is restless and anxious, difficult to console; thirsty, perhaps dry cough: *aconite 30*, Regime L.

Patient placid, weepy and wanting attention; warm and not very thirsty: *pulsatilla 30*, Regime L.

The patient is quite lively when given lots of attention, very unhappy if left alone; thirsty: *phosphorus 30*, Regime L.

Discomfort in the testes: *pulsatilla 200*, Regime A1, alongside appropriate medical attention.

If symptoms are severe or persisting too long, and other remedies are not helping: *jaborandi 30*, Regime A1.

Prevention

If a child has been in contact with someone with mumps, most homoeopaths believe that the best course is to allow the immune response to proceed naturally. However, if for some reason it is wished to do all possible to prevent it occurring at this time: *parotidinum 30*, Regime K (see *nosodes*, p. 197).

NAIL PROBLEMS

Infections under or around the nails: *silica 30*, Regime A.

Painful injuries involving the nails: *hypericum 30*, Regime B1.

Weak, brittle nails, in slightly-built individuals: *silica 12*, Regime F1.

Weak, brittle nails, in well-built individuals: *graphities 12*, Regime F1.

Constitutional treatment

To have misshapen or problem nails is a characteristic feature of several constitutional types, especially *graphities* and *thuja* but also *antim crud* and *silica*. See them in the remedy section and if one is appropriate: that remedy potency 12, Regime F1. Otherwise, a homoeopath may be able to help.

NAUSEA AND VOMITING
(Also see Stomach Pain; Nausea and Vomiting in Pregnancy)

From spoiled food
Nausea or vomiting; perhaps with diarrhoea; probably as a result of eating something spoiled; perhaps chilly and shivery; thirsty; anxious and restless state of mind; nausea and vomiting in travellers: *arsen alb 30*, Regime B1.
Nausea or vomiting; probably as a result of eating something spoiled, especially seafood; a lot of wind; craving for air; skin cool and pale perhaps even bluish: *carbo veg 30*, Regime B1.

From overindulgence
Nausea or vomiting after a binge or overindulgence; feeling irritable and oversensitive to everything; hangover: *nux vomica 30*, Regime B1.
Nausea or vomiting after a binge or overindulgence; flatulence and bloating; discomfort temporarily relieved by passing wind; feeling heavy and tired: *carbo veg 30*, Regime B1.

Motion (travel) sickness
To treat and prevent travel sickness: *cocculus 30*, Regime B1, starting one hour before setting off.

Other cases
Constant vomiting or severe nausea not relieved by vomiting: *ipecac 200*, Regime D.
Nausea or vomiting; perhaps with diarrhoea or burning pains in stomach or abdomen; anxious, restless state of mind; perhaps chilly; thirsty: *arsen alb 30*, Regime B3.
Nausea or vomiting; perhaps cramping pains in stomach or abdomen;

maybe high temperature but chilly; constantly putting on and taking off the covers; perhaps with urge to pass stool but unable to do so; or with backache: *nux vomica 30*, Regime B3.

Nausea or vomiting; perhaps with diarrhoea; thirsty; perhaps with fever or chill; patient wants constant company and reassurance to which they respond well: *phosphorus 30*, Regime B3.

Nausea or vomiting; weepy, placid state of mind and will not be left alone; thirstless; wants coolness and fresh air: *pulsatilla 30*, Regime B3.

Severe nausea or vomiting; no obvious cause; high temperature; flu-like aches in limbs; patient confused; protracted case of vomiting and diarrhoea in travellers: *baptisia 200*, Regime B3.

Constitutional treatment

A tendency to repeated attacks of nausea and vomiting needs constitutional treatment, to which such conditions generally respond well. See the constitutional remedy finder for suggestions. If a remedy is clearly indicated: that remedy potency 200, Regime C between episodes. Otherwise see a homoeopath.

NAUSEA AND VOMITING IN PREGNANCY (MORNING SICKNESS)

Constant nausea, not relieved by being sick: *ipecac 30*, Regime B1.

Nausea slightly better for eating something; cannot stand the smell of food; irritable, weepy, desire to be left alone; better for vigorous movement: *sepia 30*, Regime B1.

Nausea or vomiting; perhaps with constipation; irritable and nasty temper; chilly; better for warmth and quiet: *nux vomica 30*, Regime B1.

Nausea or vomiting; weepy and placid; need for company; better for fresh air and gentle exercise; thirstless: *pulsatilla 30*, Regime B1.

Individualised treatment

If none of the above are effective or appropriate, there are many other remedies that could help with this condition. It is recommended to consult a homoeopath.

NERVOUS DISORDERS
(Also see Fits, Convulsions, Epilepsy; Memory Loss)

This heading covers such conditions as tremors, twitches, numbness, loss of nervous control, paralysis, neurological degeneration, multiple sclerosis and Parkinson's disease.

Uncontrollable twitches, tics or spasms, perhaps particularly of the eyelids; or awkward, clumsy movements, perhaps with numbness; overexcited, impulsive state of mind; the spine sore and sensitive to touch: *agaricus 30*, Regime F2.

Twitches, uncontrollable restlessness, particularly of the legs at night; jerking movements that interrupt sleep; or a history of such followed by or combined with gradual paralysis and perhaps mental degeneration; the patient suddenly looks old; discontented state of mind: *zinc met 30*, Regime F2.

Paralysis, twitches or loss of control in any muscle group, developing gradually in intense, sympathetic individuals; perhaps after a grief or a history of morbid compulsion to constantly recheck things; or history of arthritis and contraction of tendons: *causticum 30*, Regime F2.

Degeneration of mental faculties and nervous control, heaviness of limbs leading to numbness and paralysis; intense confusion, even as to where and who one is; the patient is distressed if anyone tries to hurry him or her along; dryness of mucous skin and mucous membranes; constipation: *alumina 30*, Regime F2.

Increasing paralysis or numbness, or numbness with pain; the affected parts become weak or emaciated—hence, for example, wrist-drop; mentally slow and dull; miserable and apathetic; perhaps history of hedonistic selfindulgence: *plumbum 30*, Regime F2.

Nervous disorders where restlessness alternates with near-paralysis, mental indifference with intense activity; complete numbness, even of conditions that are normally painful; perhaps after intense fright, or shame: *opium 30*, Regime F2.

Numbness or paralysis; in affectionate, open individuals, or those once so, now increasingly withdrawn and reserved; perhaps after fright or shock or excessive stimulation; lightly-built, chilly: *phosphorus 30* Regime F2.

Constitutional and individualised treatment

Many of the conditions outlined above develop from or into constitutional states. See the constitutional remedy finder for more suggestions. If a remedy is well indicated: that remedy potency 30, Regime F2. If none of the above are appropriate or effective, consult a homoeopath, which in general is highly advisable.

NIGHTMARES
(Also see Sleeplessness)

Nightmares that begin after a particular shock or fright: *aconite 200*, Regime A2 (at bedtime).
After grief or bereavement: *ignatia 200*, Regime A2 (at bedtime).
After a protracted period of disturbing experiences: *opium 200*, Regime A2 (at bedtime).
In sensitive, affectionate, imaginative, impressionable people, especially children: *phosphorus 200*, Regime A2 (at bedtime).
In inquisitive, boisterous people, especially children: *sulphur 200*, Regime A2 (at bedtime).

Constitutional treatment

If none of the above help, constitutional treatment may do so, especially if the nightmares are a feature of wider psychological or behavioural issues. *Anacardium*, *hyoscyamus*, *natrum mur*, *nux vomica* and *stramonium* are among the other remedy types that might be predisposed to this kind of difficulty. See them in the remedy section, and see the constitutional remedy finder for suggestions. If a remedy is clearly indicated: that remedy potency 200, Regime A2. Otherwise see a homoeopath.

NOSEBLEEDS

After a blow or injury (or picking): *arnica 30*, Regime I.
Spontaneous flow of bright red blood: *ipecac 30*, Regime I.
Nosebleed during cough or fever: *phosphorus 30*, Regime B3.
During dry, violent coughing fits, if *phosphorus* does not work: *drosera 30*, Regime B3.
If the nose continues to bleed slowly for a long time: *hamamelis 30*, Regime D.

Constitutional treatment

A tendency to recurrent nosebleeds often responds well to constitutional treatment. *China*, *lachesis* and *phosphorus* types are prone to them. Consider them in the remedy section, and see the constitutional remedy finder for more suggestions. If a remedy is well indicated: that remedy potency 30, Regime I during bleeds, and potency 200, Regime C between them. Otherwise, see a homoeopath.

OBESITY

To stimulate the thyroid gland, tone up the metabolism and thus accelerate weight-loss during diet and other adjustments to lifestyle: *fucus ves* (kelp) *mother tincture*, Regime E2.
If *fucus* is ineffective: *phytolacca mother tincture*, Regime E2.

Constitutional treatment

Constitutional treatment can help with emotional, hormonal and metabolic conditions that may be partly responsible for excessive weight. It cannot change a person's basic body-type.

It is certainly worth seeking homoeopathic treatment for help and support if one is going to make determined efforts at dieting and exercise. *Antim crud*, *calc carb*, *ferrum met* and *graphities* are among the types most prone to obesity. *Calc carb*, *kali carb*, *lycopodium* and *sulphur* are some of the types with a tendency to sugar craving. *Natrum mur* and *carbo veg* love salt. *Natrum mur* and *sulphur* desire starchy things. Consider those remedies in the remedy section, and see the constitutional remedy finder for more suggestions. If a remedy is clearly indicated: that remedy potency 30. Otherwise consult a homoeopath.

OPERATIONS

The remedies below can be taken together if more than one is appropriate (which is often the case). Specialist homoeopathic pharmacies will prepare them combined if necessary, to make them as simple as possible to take in hospital. The remedies will still be effective if the patient is receiving any conventional medication, with which they will not interfere in any way.

Remedies to be taken internally

To minimise discomfort, bleeding and bruising; protect against shock and infection; and to promote the healing process after any operation: *arnica 200*, Regime H3.

Operations to the spine, head, fingers, toes, dental roots and any parts rich in nerves: *hypericum 200*, Regime H3.

Surgical procedures involving deep incisions that remain uncomfortable for long periods; particularly to the pelvic organs and genitals, including episiotomies, caesarian sections and hysterectomies; also for the psychological parallels of deep cuts: *staphisagria 200*, Regime H3.

Surgical procedures that involve deep incisions particularly to the abdominal and pelvic organs; also operations to the breast, including lumpectomies; to minimise discomfort and promote healing: *bellis perennis 200*, Regime H3.

Any surgical procedures in which bones are to be broken, reset, grafted or passed through, including cosmetic operations: *sympthytum 30*, Regime H3. (If there are going to be multiple operations, do not start taking this remedy until the bones have been restored to the position in which they are to heal.)

Operations to veins, varicosities and the anus: *hamamelis 200*, Regime H3.

Operations on tendons, ligaments and cartilage (including the accommodation of the eye): *ruta 200*, Regime H3.

Operations, including cosmetic surgery, to or around the eye, to further reduce bruising and promote healing: *ledum 200*, Regime H3 (alongside *arnica*).

Wherever much skin or flesh is to be cut or denuded, to promote the regrowth of tissues and to minimise scarring: *calendula 30*, Regime H.

Local applications

Apply to uncovered wounds that are delicate and tender: *hypericum and calendula mother tinctures*, Regime N.

To narrow incisions and partly-healed wounds: *hypericum and calendula cream*, Regime M.

To bruised areas (but not to the incisions): *arnica cream*, Regime M.

OSTEOPOROSIS: see Bone Degeneration, p. 29.

PELVIC INFLAMMATORY DISEASE

For attacks of cystitis or period problems, see those sections. Otherwise, PID itself needs constitutional treatment to raise health and resistance generally. *Cannabis, medorrhinum, mercurius* and *thuja* types are among those prone to this kind of problem. Consider them in the remedy section, and see the constitutional remedy finder for more suggestions. If a remedy is clearly indicated: that remedy potency 200, Regime C. Otherwise, you are advised to consult a homoeopath.

PERIOD PROBLEMS
(Also see Periods Delayed; Female Reproductive System)

Mood changes before periods, pms
Intense irritability, cannot resist cutting and unkind remarks; craving to be alone; averse to any touch; sudden tears; perhaps headache: *sepia 30*, Regime B.
Vicious irritability, sense of being surrounded by fools; oversensitive to noise and imperfections; perhaps craving coffee or other stimulants which actually make things worse; perhaps constipation: *nux vomica 30*, Regime B.
Tearful and cross by turns; wishing for really kind and supportive company; perhaps cross with oneself for feeling needy; cannot bear lack of fresh air: *pulsatilla 30*, Regime B.
Irritable about small things, sad about big ones; resentful; upset about things that happened a long time ago; dry skin and greasy hair; perhaps headaches: *natrum mur 30*, Regime B.
Foul, capricious, childish bad temper: *chamomilla 200*, Regime B.
And see the note on constitutional treatment, p. 93.

Dysmenorrhoea, painful periods
Cutting, twisting pains; some relief from curling up and particularly from pressure; pains felt particularly in the ovaries; better from heat: *colocynth 30*, Regime B1.
Pain in sudden neuralgic spasms; better for curling up and pressure; some improvement when the flow starts; better for heat: *mag phos 30*, Regime B1.
Pains better when the flow starts; pain extends to the back; bright

red bleeding; clotting; feeling hot and rather wild-headed or giddy: *belladonna 30*, Regime B1.

Cramping, griping pain; pains better for heat; clotting; very irritable and capricious: *chamomilla 30*, Regime B1.

General soreness of whole pelvic area; steady flow of dark blood: *hamamelis 30*, Regime B1.

Pain in sudden neuralgic spasms; better for heat; better for keeping still; worse for pressure; short-tempered and nasty mood: *nux vomica 30*, Regime B1.

Cramping or dragging pains; better for curling up or moving around in the fresh air; clotting; flow intermittent; tearful, in need of supportive company: *pulsatilla 30*, Regime B1.

Dragging pains as if parts would prolapse; pain extending to the back and thighs; flow intermittent; generally chilly; tearful and irritable; averse to company: *sepia 30*, Regime B1.

And see the note on constitutional treatment, p. 93.

Heavy periods, menorrhagia
Profuse, steady flow of rather dark blood: *hamamelis 30*, Regime B.
Gushes of bright red blood: *ipecac 30*, Regime B1.
Profuse, clotted blood: *sabina 30*, Regime B.
Weakness after loss of much blood: *china 30*, Regime A.
And see the note on constitutional treatment, p. 93.

Bleeding between periods
With abdominal pain or severe irritability: *chamomilla 30*, Regime B.
Profuse, bright red blood: *ipecac 30*, Regime B.
In slightly-built, affectionate, impressionable, chilly individuals: *phosphorus 30*, Regime B.
If none of the above apply: *sabina 30*, Regime B.
And see the note on constitutional treatment, p. 93.

Periods absent, amenorrhea
From loss of sleep, disturbance of the body-clock: *cocculus 30*, Regime B.
From recent emotional distress, grief or disappointment: *ignatia 30*, Regime A.
From emotional distress, grief or disappointment over six weeks ago: *nat mur 200*, Regime C.
After a bad shock or fright: *opium 200*, Regime C.

After a debilitating illness, especially if much fluid was lost, with anaemia: *china 30*, Regime A.
And see the note on constitutional treatment below.

Constitutional and individualised treatment

If none of the suggestions above are appropriate or effective, constitutional treatment will help a lot in many cases. See the constitutional
remedy finder for suggestions. If a remedy is clearly indicated: that
remedy potency 30, Regime B during episodes, and potency 200,
Regime C between them. Otherwise consult a homoeopath.

PERIODS DELAYED

This needs and often responds well to constitutional treatment. See the
baryta carb, *calc carb*, *phosphorus*, *pulsatilla* and *silica* types as
described in the remedy section. If one of them is clearly indicated:
that remedy potency 200, Regime C. Otherwise consult a homoeopath.

Nosebleeds
If the girl is getting lots of nosebleeds, consider *phosphorus* particularly
carefully and also *pulsatilla* and *silica*. If none of them is appropriate
or effective: *bryonia 200*, Regime C.

PILES, HAEMORRHOIDS

Piles that come up occasionally, after straining at stool, or with bleeding
and soreness; often external: *hamamelis 30*, Regime B1.
Piles, little or no bleeding, severe pain as if the rectum were full of
sharp things; perhaps with backache, worse for sitting, standing and
walking; protrude during stool; perhaps during pregnancy: *aesculus
30*, Regime A.
Piles, little or no bleeding, not large, but very painful; perhaps during
period or pregnancy: *collinsonia 30*, Regime A.
Piles in irritable, impatient, chilly individuals; perhaps worse after a
binge or much indulgence; pain worse for touch or pressure; perhaps
with constipation or during pregnancy: *nux vomica 30*, Regime A.
Piles that itch or burn, often external, discomfort worse for standing or
walking and for touch or pressure; perhaps with moisture from anus;
perhaps during menopause or after childbirth: *sulphur 30*, Regime A.

Discomfort relieved by slow walking and cool applications; patient tearful or placid, perhaps with moisture from the anus, perhaps during period or pregnancy: *pulsatilla 30*, Regime A.

After childbirth; perhaps with demanding and bad-tempered moods; chilly; perhaps with backache: *kali carb 30*, Regime A.

Constitutional and individualised treatment

If none of the above is appropriate or effective, and for long-term tendencies to this problem, constitutional treatment is needed. Many of the possibilities outlined above may develop from or into constitutional conditions. Other types prone to piles include *arsenicum*, *graphities*, *lachesis* (particularly around times of hormonal changes), *lycopodium*, *nitric acid*, *phosphorus* and *sepia* (also around times of hormonal changes). Consider those remedies as described in the remedy section of this book, and see the constitutional remedy finder for more suggestions. If a remedy is clearly indicated: that remedy potency 30, Regime A during attacks, or potency 200, Regime C between them. Otherwise consult a homoeopath.

Local applications
Creams or suppositories containing *aesculus* or *hamamelis*, or both, may provide some relief at least in the short-term, and can be used alongside internal remedies.

PRICKLY HEAT, SUN REACTIONS

Red patches or itchy red spots: *urtica 30*, Regime B1.
Angry red spots, perhaps like blisters, more stinging than itching: *apis 30*, Regime B1.

Local application
Urtica cream, Regime M, or *urtica mother tincture*, Regime N.

Prevention
To reduce sensitivity to the sun: *sol 30*, Regime F5. (This may seem unlikely, but a significant number of people have reported good results.)

PROSTATE ENLARGEMENT

Classic symptoms of prostate enlargement, must wait for urine to flow: *sabal serr 2X*, Regime F2.
If *sabal serr* is not effective: *chimaphila 2X*, Regime F2.

Constitutional treatment

If the above do not help, constitutional treatment will do so in at least a significant number of cases. *Calc carb*, *lycopodium* and *pulsatilla* types are particularly prone to this problem. Consider them in the remedy section, and see the constitutional remedy finder for more suggestions. If a remedy is clearly indicated: that remedy potency 30, Regime A. Otherwise consult a homoeopath.

PSORIASIS

Classic psoriasis; silvery flakes over red, sore skin; in slightly-built, warm-blooded, active individuals: *arsen iod 200*, Regime C.
No clear indications for any remedy: *morgan co 200*, Regime C.

Constitutional treatment

Psoriasis can be a difficult and stubborn condition to resolve, even for experienced homoeopaths, and in a substantial number of cases it yields at least partially to one of the remedies above without clear indications, when all else seems to have failed. None the less, constitutional treatment is usually the best course. *Graphities*, *lycopodium*, *sepia*, *staphisagria* and *sulphur* types are among those most prone to the problem. Consider them in the remedy section, and see the constitutional remedy finder for suggestions. If a remedy is clearly indicated: that remedy potency 30, Regime A during attacks, or potency 200, Regime C between them. Otherwise consult a homoeopath.

RECTUM, BLEEDING
(Also see Bowels and Colon Problems; Piles)

Occasional slight bleeding, particularly after passing an unusually large or hard stool: *hamamelis 30*, Regime A.
Passing much blood, perhaps with known tendency to ulcerations, or

during a fever or gastroenteritis, particularly during or after travel to unfamiliar places: *merc corr 30*, Regime A.

Some blood in the stool, during illness, with burning pains and perhaps fever; worse at night and for cold things; anxious mood, difficult to reassure: *arsen alb 30*, Regime B1.

Some blood in the stool, during illness, perhaps with fever; worse in the evening and for hot food; anxious mood, needs light and company, the patient responds to reassurance: *phosphorus 30*, Regime B1.

Constitutional treatment

Once the appropriate clinical investigations have been carried out, stubborn or recurrent rectal bleeding needs constitutional treatment, to which it generally responds well, whether or not diverticulitis, haemorrhoids, or any other conditions have been diagnosed.

Among the types most prone to this sort of problem are *argent nit*, *arsenicum*, *nitric acid*, *phosphorus* and *sulphur*. See them in the remedy section, and consult the constitutional remedy finder for more suggestions. If a remedy is well-indicated: that remedy potency 30, Regime A during attacks, or potency 200, Regime C between them. Otherwise it is best to see a homoeopath.

RUBELLA: see German Measles, p. 62.

SCIATICA

Specific remedies

Pain worse at rest and starting to move, better with continued motion, better walking; worse cold and particularly in damp and cold conditions; worse lying on the back or on the affected side; perhaps with numbness: *rhus tox 200*, Regime B.

Pain much worse when cold, and hence from uncovering, better heat and much better pressure, hence better lying on the affected side; perhaps worse on the right side; pains come and go suddenly: *mag phos 200*, Regime B.

Pain worse with motion, much worse walking; worse on the left side; pain in successive shocks; perhaps from hip to ankle; better heat; direct pressure to the pain is worse, but lying on the affected side feels better; perhaps with numbness: *colocynth 200*, Regime B.

Sciatica after injuries to the legs or back, sharp cutting pains along the
course of the nerve, worse sitting, perhaps worse on the left side:
hypericum 200, Regime B.

Constitutional and individualised treatment

Often what is needed for sciatica is a constitutional remedy, both for
the tendency to get the problem and frequently for the pains when they
happen. There are also many other remedies that may be helpful for
the pains, which a trained homoeopath could consider. Among the types
prone to sciatica are *arsen alb, lachesis, lycopodium, nux vomica,* and
pulsatilla. See them in the remedy section, and consult the constitutional
remedy finder for more suggestions. If one is well indicated: that remedy
potency 30, Regime B1 during attacks, or potency 200, Regime C
between them. Otherwise, see a homoeopath.

SEXUAL PROBLEMS

Lack of desire, impotence, in men
Strong desire but complete impotence, after excessive sexual activity
or alcohol; with general physical and mental prostration: *selenium
30*, Regime F2.
High sex drive but with incomplete erections or premature ejaculation:
conium 30, Regime F2.
Impotence after grief, long illness or depression, with general physical
weakness and mental indifference: *phosphoric acid 30*, Regime F2.
Loss of sexual desire in previously sexually active men: *agnus cast 30*,
Regime F2.
Easily excited but erection incomplete; the more one feels responsible
or committed to the partner, the worse it seems to be: *lycopodium
200*, Regime C.
And see the note on constitutional treatment, p. 98.

Lack of desire, aversion to sex, in women
(Also see Vaginal Problems)
Loss of sexual desire without obvious cause in previously sexually
active women: *agnus cast 30*, Regime F2.
Lack of desire after grief, long illness or depression, with general physi-
cal weakness and mental indifference: *phosphoric acid 30*, Regime
F2.

Feeling put-upon, harassed, used but unappreciated, great aversion to being touched, longing to be left alone: *sepia 200*, Regime C.
And see the note on constitutional treatment below.

Excessive sexual desire
Not relieved after intercourse: *cantharis 30*, Regime F2.
And see the note on constitutional treatment below.

Constitutional and individualised treatment

If none of the above is effective, constitutional treatment will help in a significant proportion of cases. Homoeopathy cannot 'cure' reduced desire at times such as after childbirth, or declining sexual vigour with advancing age, when it would be natural and beneficial for the energies to be invested elsewhere. Neither can it resolve or change what one really does and does not desire, although it can often help with any necessary emotional adjustments. Constitutional treatment may help if sexual precocity is a feature of behavioural problems in children.

Remedy types prone to impotence in men include *baryta carb* and *lycopodium*. Types prone to long-term loss of desire or aversion to sex in women include *causticum*, *lycopodium*, *natrum mur* and *sepia*. Among the types prone to problematically high sex drive are *cantharis*, *cannabis*, *hyoscyamus*, *medorrhinum*, *platina* and *tuberculinum*. Emotional difficulties relating to sex are common among *hyoscyamus*, *natrum mur*, *mercurius*, *staphisagria* and *thuja* types.

Consider those remedies in the remedy section and see the constitutional remedy finder for more suggestions. If one is well indicated: that remedy potency 200, Regime C. Otherwise consult a homoeopath. (It is reasonable to expect a homoeopath to be willing to invest a little time in a preliminary discussion, perhaps by phone, to establish if treatment might be helpful in the case and if the necessary rapport can be established between homoeopath and patient.)

SHINGLES (HERPES ZOSTER)

Small red blisters; intense itching or burning pains; some relief from heat and moving around: *rhus tox 200*, Regime A1.
Burning and intense itching; eruptions are dark red or even bluish; pains

worse for being touched and moving around; usually affects mature individuals: *ranunculus 200*, Regime A1.

Severe burning pains; especially if eruptions discharge pus or serum that forms crusts; especially if scalp is affected; usually affects mature individuals: *mezereum 200*, Regime A1.

Burning pains, relieved by heat, the patient is chilly, fussy, anxious and restless: *arsen alb 200*, Regime A1.

Shingles around the eyes: *ranunculus 200*, Regime A1.

Pains after shingles; post-herpetic neuralgia: *mezereum 200*, Regime A1.

Pains after shingles, *mezereum* does not help: *hypericum 200*, Regime A1.

Supplementary remedy to be given alongside any of the above throughout treatment: *herpes zoster nosode 200*, Regime A2.

Supplementary remedy to be given alongside any of the above throughout treatment if shingles occurred after contact with chicken pox (instead of herpes nosode): *varicella 200*, Regime A2.

Local application
To sooth the skin and prevent infection if eruptions break: *hypericum and calendula mother tincture*, Regime N.

Constitutional and individualised treatment

Stubborn or recurrent cases may respond to constitutional treatment. As well as those mentioned above, *graphities*, *lachesis*, *mercurius*, *natrum mur*, *sulphur* and *thuja* types are prone to the problem. See them in the remedy section, and consult the constitutional remedy finder for more suggestions. If a remedy is clearly indicated: that remedy potency 30, Regime A1 during attacks. Otherwise consult a homoeopath.

SHOCK AND FRIGHT
(Also see Collapse, Fainting; Fear and Anxiety)

Person injured, suffering from shock: *arnica 200*, Regime D. If medical attention is required: Regime G.

The immediate effects of a shock or fright that has just happened: *aconite 200*, Regime D.

Symptoms which definitely began after a shock or fright that happened some time ago; these could be physical symptoms such as missed periods or digestive upsets or anything else, or occasional panic attacks with great fear: *aconite 1M*, Regime C.

The aftermath of a shock or fright involving violence or horrors; bad dreams, terrors, a disturbed and rather manic state of mind, perhaps afraid of the dark and being alone: *stramonium 200*, Regime C.

The aftermath of a shock or fright, with numbness, stupefaction or hopelessness, perhaps alternating with periods of fear or a peculiar sense of well-being: *opium 200*, Regime C.

Individualised and constitutional treatment

Apart from the suggestions above, the effects of shock or fright could require any of a great number of possible remedies. *Argent nit*, *hyoscyamus*, *opium*, *phosphorus* and *stramonium* are among the remedies most often indicated in such situations. Consider them in the remedy section, and see the constitutional remedy finder for more suggestions. If a remedy is clearly indicated: that remedy potency 200, Regime C. Otherwise consult a homoeopath.

SINUSITIS

Symptoms a little better for fresh air and much worse in stuffy places; if there is a discharge it is thick, yellow, green or white catarrh; perhaps with disagreeable subjective smell in the nose; perhaps placid or weepy state of mind: *pulsatilla 30*, Regime A1.

Thick catarrh which is stringy and difficult to be rid of; yellow or green; pain in the sinuses concentrated in certain points: *kali bich 30*, Regime A1.

Thick, yellow mucus; sinuses feel raw and sore; catarrh flows more when outside: *hydrastis 30*, Regime A1.

Pain in the sinuses with profuse watery discharge from the nose; the patient feels hot, symptoms better for fresh air: *kali iod 30*, Regime A1.

Profuse post-natal drip, none of the above particularly apply: *corallium rub 30*, Regime A1.

Long-standing cases; little or no discharge: *silica 200*, Regime A3.

Constitutional and individualised treatment

For stubborn or recurrent sinusitis constitutional treatment is needed. *Kali bich*, *lycopodium*, *mercurius*, *medorrhinum*, *pulsatilla*, *thuja* and *silica* types are prone to the problem. Consider them in the remedy section, and see the constitutional remedy finder for more suggestions. If a remedy is clearly indicated: that remedy potency 30, Regime A1 during attacks, or potency 200, Regime C between them. Otherwise consult a homoeopath.

SLEEPLESSNESS
(Also see Nightmares)

After a severe shock or fright: *aconite 1M*, Regime C.
From recent grief, loss or disappointment: *ignatia 200*, Regime A2 (take on retiring).
From grief, loss or disappointment, more than six weeks ago: *natrum mur 1M*, Regime C.
From general overactivity of the mind, not unhappy, just unable to switch off; or from excitement before a happy event; or if rather tense and oversensitive to slight sounds: *coffea 30*, Regime H5.
From anxiety before an ordeal like an exam: *aconite 30*, Regime H5.
From anxiety, in thin-built, conscientious types: *arsen alb 200*, Regime A2 (take on retiring).
After hard work, cannot stop thinking of it; concerned about details; irritable; sleeplessness perhaps aggravated by use of stimulants; especially if one tends to wake at about 4 a.m.: *nux vomica 30*, Regime H5.
After childbirth: *coffea 200*, Regime A2 (take on retiring).
From disturbance of the body-clock after night-watching, jet-lag or change of shifts: *cocculus 200*, Regime A2 (take on retiring).
If nothing else works: *passiflora mother tincture*, Regime E4.

Constitutional treatment

Chronic sleeplessness needs constitutional treatment, although this is not an easy condition to treat. *Arsen alb*, *carcinosin*, *coffea*, *lachesis* and *phosphorus* types are among those most prone to it. Sleeplessness in refined, conscientious children is very characteristic of *carcinosin*. Consider them, and see the constitutional remedy finder for more suggestions. If a remedy is clearly indicated: that remedy potency 200, Regime A2 (take on retiring).

SPLEEN PROBLEMS

If malfunction of the spleen has been diagnosed, to be taken alongside constitutional treatment and appropriate clinical measures: *ceanothus mother tincture*, Regime E.

SPLINTERS

Deep, small splinters that cannot be removed, to promote expulsion: *silica 200*, Regime A3.
If the area around the splinter becomes sore or infected: *hepar sulph 30*, Regime A1.

Local application
Once the splinter has been removed, to prevent infection and promote healing: *hypericum and calendula mother tincture*, Regime N2, or *cream*, Regime M.

STOMACH PAIN, INDIGESTION, ACIDITY
(Also see Nausea and Vomiting; Ulcers, Stomach; Abdominal Pain)

Straightforward occasional indigestion
Indigestion after overeating or eating too quickly, food sitting like a lump in the stomach; pains tend to come on some time after eating; perhaps with ineffectual belching; perhaps nauseous; bad-tempered; also tummy ache in irritable children: *nux vomica 30*, Regime B2.
Indigestion from overeating or unsuitable food, during or just after eating; burning or acidic pains; perhaps nauseous; anxious moods; also tummy ache in anxious children: *arsen abl 30*, Regime B2.
Indigestion from eating fatty or creamy food; perhaps nauseous; craving fresh air; also tummy ache in clingy children: *pulsatilla 30*, Regime B2.
Pain comes on during or just after eating; and particularly in the late afternoon; much flatulence passing downwards; pains tend to be worse on the right side; symptoms worse before an important event: *lycopodium 30*, Regime B1.

Indigestion from overeating or unsuitable food; bloated with lots of wind; feeling heavy and lethargic: *carbo veg 30*, Regime B2.

Recurrent stomach pains and disorders

These conditions require constitutional treatment. Some of the constitutional types most prone to them include *anacardium* (pains better for eating; in discontented individuals); *antim crud* (pains with thick-coated tongue; sentimental moods); *arsen alb* (burning pains; anxious, fastidious individuals); *china* (with bloating, in refined individuals); *lycopodium* (pains come on in the late afternoon, worse on the right side); *nux vomica* (urge to burp or vomit but cannot; irritable mood); *phosphorus* (worse for hot food; gregarious individuals); *sulphur* (worse fatty foods, worse standing).

See them in the remedy section, and consult the constitutional remedy finder for more suggestions. If one fits well: that remedy potency 30, Regime B2 during attacks, or potency 200, Regime C between them. Otherwise consult a homoeopath. This sort of problem generally responds well to accurate prescribing, even if ulceration or other conditions are becoming established, and effective treatment can avoid more serious developments.

STRAINS AND SPRAINS
(Also see Arthritis and Rheumatism)

Recent injuries
If medical attention is required: *arnica 200*, Regime G.
If the accident or injury has just happened and it is not yet clear what damage has been done: *arnica 200*, Regime D.
If the pain is particularly severe when the part is moved and arnica does not help: *bryonia 200*, Regime D.

Established cases
Stiffness and pain that is worse when the affected part is first moved but which eases with continued motion. Better with warmth: *rhus tox 30*, Regime B.
If pain does not vary much with movement, and the injured part feels too weak to bear weight: *ruta 30*, Regime B.
Old injuries (more than six weeks) where nothing else is helping: *strontium carb 30*, Regime A.

STRESS, INNER TENSION
(Also see Anger; Fear and Anxiety; Depression; Grief; Sleeplessness)

Too much to do, too little time, surrounded by fools: *nux vomica 30*, Regime A.

Because there are so many things that will go wrong if one is not really careful: *arsen alb 30*, Regime A.

Because so many people want things, and they never leave you in peace: *sepia 30*, Regime A.

Because people are so rude, disrespectful and inconsiderate: *staphisagria 30*, Regime A.

Constitutional treatment

Just as all personality types can suffer inner tension, so absolutely any homoeopathic remedy might be needed for a particular case. See the constitutional remedy finder for suggestions. If one is well indicated: that remedy potency 30, Regime A. Otherwise see a homoeopath.

STROKE

Suspected or threatened stroke: *carbo veg 200*, Regime G.

Suspected or threatened stroke; patient very frightened: *aconite 200*, Regime G.

Suspected or threatened stroke; patient loses consciousness: *opium 200*, Regime G.

Immediately after a stroke to promote recovery: *arnica 6* and *kali mur 6*, both Regime H1.

After a stroke, if the patient has lost all interest in things, just sits and stares into space: *carbo animalis 30*, Regime F6.

After a stroke, if there is loss of short-term memory, symptoms of childishness or senility: *baryta carb 30*, Regime F6.

After a stroke, if the main symptoms are vertigo and disorientation; placid state of mind: *cocculus 30*, Regime F6.

After a stroke, patient is weak, shaky, dizzy and sleepy: *gelsemium 30*, Regime F6.

After a stroke, the patient is aware of his or her situation and deeply depressed: *aurum 30*, Regime F6.

Individualised treatment

If none of the above is effective or appropriate, individualised treatment is needed, taking into consideration the present symptoms and the nature of the patient before the stroke occurred. You are recommended to consult a homoeopath.

SUNSTROKE, HYPERTHERMIA, OVERHEATING

If medical attention is required: *belladonna 200*, Regime G.

Bright red skin, bounding pulse, dilated pupils or rather wild eyes, pulsating pains and headaches, perhaps not much sweat, especially after falling asleep in the sun; dizziness or disorientation: *belladonna 200*, Regime B2.

Surges of heat and pain rising to the head; intense pounding headache; symptoms much worse for any more heat: *glonoine 200*, Regime B2.

Sudden flushes of intense heat, followed by sweating: *amyl nit 200*, Regime B2.

Ailments remaining after sunstroke a long time ago: *glonoine 1M*, Regime C.

Dehydration after overheating and prolonged sweating leaving weakness or vertigo: *china 30*, Regime A1.

TESTES PROBLEMS, ORCHITIS, EPIDIDYMITIS

Pain or swelling remains after a blow to the testicles: *arnica 200*, Regime A1.

Hardening, pain or swelling, particularly of the epididymis; better for warmth; worse before changes in the weather, perhaps worse on the right side; perhaps personal or family history of sexual conditions: *rhododendron 30*, Regime A.

Pain or hardening of testes or epididymis; pain worse for heat in bed; worse at night; perhaps personal or family history of sexual conditions: *clematis 30*, Regime A.

Pain or swelling of testes or epididymis; worse for heat, perhaps worse left side; patient placid or tearful; orchitis during or after childhood illnesses: *pulsatilla 30,* Regime A1.

Pain in testes after sexual stimulation without discharge: *staphisagria 30*, Regime B2.

Testes become very hard, and maybe swollen, perhaps after forced or voluntary celibacy: *conium 30*, Regime A.

Aching, swelling or hardening of the testicles, worse on the right side, during or after a period of deep unhappiness: *aurum 200*, Regime C.

Constitutional treatment

In long-term and recurrent cases, constitutional treatment is needed. *Argent nit, aurum, medorrhinum, pulsatilla, staphisagria* and *thuja* are among the types prone to this kind of problem. See them in the remedy section, and consult the constitutional remedy finder for more suggestions. If a remedy is well indicated: that remedy potency 30, Regime A1 during attacks, or potency 200 between them. Otherwise consult a homoeopath. Good treatment can help much in these conditions and avoid the development of more serious problems.

TESTICLES, UNDESCENDED

Undescended testicle in plump, warm-blooded, mild-tempered, rather weepy or clingy boys: *pulsatilla 200*, Regime C.

Neither testicle descended in rather skinny, undeveloped boys: *aurum 200*, Regime C.

Right testicle not descended, in rather serious, self-conscious boys: *lycopodium 200*, Regime C.

Right testicle not descended; family history of sexual conditions: *clematis 200*, Regime C.

Nothing else is appropriate: *thyroidinum 200*, Regime C.

Individualised treatment

If none of the above is effective, consult a homoeopath.

THROAT, SORE, INFECTIONS, TONSILLITIS
(Also see Voice Lost)

Sore throat, just come on, symptoms developing quickly, perhaps been chilled or feeling feverish: *aconite 30*, Regime B3.

Sore throat, just come on, symptoms developing slowly, few other symptoms, perhaps slightly feverish or tired: *ferrum phos 30*, Regime B1.

Sore throat, some fever, slightly dizzy; perhaps started or worse on the right side; perhaps tonsils inflamed: *belladonna 30*, Regime B1.

Sore throat, feelings like the first symptoms of 'flu: *gelsemium 30*, Regime B1.

Sore throat, perhaps tonsillitis; perhaps with pockets of pus; unpleasant, metallic taste in the mouth; salivating more than usual; symptoms get worse at night: *mercurius 30*, Regime B1.

Sore throat or swollen tonsils, worse on the left side or started left and moved right; pains worse when swallowing liquids and especially when swallowing nothing, swallowing food is not so bad; worse for heat, better cool things: *lachesis 30*, Regime B1.

Worse on the right or started right to left; worse for cold things; symptoms worse in late afternoon: *lycopodium 30*, Regime B1.

Sore throat or tonsillitis; perhaps with pockets of pus; pains much worse for cold things and better heat; generally chilly and very irritable: *hepar sulph 30*, Regime B1.

Sore throat or swollen tonsils; worse for hot drinks; pain extends to the ear; perhaps glands of neck and under chin swollen and sore: *phytolacca 30*, Regime B1.

Nothing else clearly indicated, symptoms definitely worse on the right side: *merc iod flav 30*, Regime B1.

Nothing else clearly indicated, symptoms definitely worse on the left side: *merc iod rub 30*, Regime B1.

Swelling of the uvula, as if full of fluid; pains worse for heat: *apis 30*, Regime B1.

Constitutional treatment

Persistent or recurrent sore throats or tonsillitis require constitutional treatment, to which they generally respond well. Among the types prone to chronic swollen tonsils are *baryta carb*, *psorinum*, *silica* and *tuberculinum*. See them and the constitutional remedy finder for more suggestions. If one is well indicated: that remedy potency 30, Regime B1 during flare-ups, or potency 200, Regime C in between. Otherwise see a homoeopath.

THROMBOSIS

Thrombosis on the left side of the body, particularly if the affected part is at all bluish, and if the individual is warm-blooded: *lachesis 30*, Regime F2.

On the right side of the body, or in chilly, timid individuals: *bothrops 30*, Regime F2.

Constitutional treatment

Recurrent or persistent thrombosis requires constitutional treatment. *Apis, arsen alb, carbo veg, lachesis* and *natrum sulph* are among the remedies prone to this condition. See them in the remedy section. If one is well indicated: that remedy potency 30, Regime F2. In general it is best to see a homoeopath, especially if conventional drugs are being taken.

THRUSH, ORAL
(Also see Candida Albicans)

If there is smelly breath, increased salivation, tongue sore or indented: *mercurius 30*, Regime A1.

With dry mouth and skin, greasy hair, miserable mood and perhaps headaches: *natrum mur 30*, Regime A1.

In cases with few other physical or mental symptoms, especially children and mothers or babies while breast-feeding: *borax 30*, Regime A1.

Nothing else works: *hydrastis 30*, Regime A1.

Constitutional treatment

Persistent or recurrent thrush needs constitutional treatment to which it often responds well. Among the many types prone to this sort of condition are *antim crud, arsen alb, natrum phos, calc carb, pulsatilla* and *sulphur*. See them in the remedy section, and consult the constitutional remedy finder for more suggestions. If a remedy is well indicated: that remedy potency 30, Regime A1 during attacks, or potency 200, Regime C between them. Otherwise see a homoeopath.

THYROID PROBLEMS

Classic symptoms of overactive thyroid; hungry but thin, warm-blooded and worse for heat; very active and must keep busy; perhaps with hardening or swelling of thyroid glands, possibly protrusion of the eyes: *iodum 30*, Regime F2.

Underactive thyroid; little appetite but still putting on weight; chilly, lethargic; perhaps with swelling of thyroid and protrusion of eyes: *calc carb 30*, Regime F2.

Marginally underactive thyroid, tendency to put on weight: *fucus ves* (kelp) *mother tincture*, Regime E.

Thyroid problems in chilly people prone to coughs or asthma: *spongia 30*, Regime F2.

Thyroid problems, come on after emotional trauma: *natrum mur 200*, Regime C.

Constitutional and individualised treatment

If none of the above is appropriate or effective, individualised treatment is needed. *Calc carb, iodum, lycopodium, phosphorus, silica* and *spongia* types are among those most prone to this sort of problem. See them in the remedy section and if one is well indicated: that remedy potency 30, Regime F2.

A number of lesser-used remedies derived from chemical compounds with a role in metabolism are often what is really needed in cases of thyroid problems. Also the thyroid gland in homoeopathic potency (*thyroidinum*) can be helpful in both overactivity and underactivity, either alone or alongside other remedies. (A typical dose is *thyroidinum 6*, Regime F2.) And it is possible to do more if treatment is begun before regular use of thyroxine is established. For all these reasons, it is highly advisable to consult a homoeopath.

TINNITUS

During or aggravated by headaches: *china 30*, Regime B1.

With vertigo, in slightly-built, gregarious individuals: *phosphorus 30*, Regime B1.

One's own voice echoes in the ears: *causticum 200*, Regime C.

In warm-blooded, conscientious individuals: *kali iod 30*, Regime A.

Ringing or buzzing sounds, perhaps with vertigo, or if none of the other remedies are indicated: *china sulph 30*, Regime A.

Constitutional treatment

Tinnitus is not an easy condition to treat and probably responds well in less than 50 per cent of cases, but constitutional treatment is worth trying if none of the above is effective. *Calc carb*, *china*, *graphities*, *lycopodium*, *pulsatilla* and *sulphur* are among the types prone to it. See them in the remedy section, and consult the constitutional remedy finder for more suggestions. If one is well indicated: that remedy potency 30, Regime B1 during attacks, or potency 200, Regime C between them. Otherwise see a homoeopath.

TOOTH PROBLEMS
(Also see Abscesses; Gum Disease)

Toothache
Neuralgic pain in the teeth, worse for noise and any emotions: *coffea 200*, Regime B1.
Pains in the teeth, from suspected caries or no obvious cause, while waiting for dental investigation: *chamomilla 200*, Regime B1.
Pain from caries, while waiting for dental attention: *plantago 200*, Regime B1. (May usefully be taken with *chamomilla*.)
A tendency to pains in the teeth, or headaches that extend to teeth, particularly if associated with feelings of intense anger or humiliation: *staphisagria 200*, Regime B1.

Weakness of teeth or predisposition to tooth decay
In heavily-built individuals: *calc carb 6X*, Regime F4.
In thin-built, thin-chested, dry-skinned individuals or rather undeveloped children: *calc phos 6X*, Regime F4.
In individuals with the kind of body type that tends to curvature of bones and hypermobility of joints: *calc fluor 6X*, Regime F4.

Constitutional treatment

A recurrent tendency to pain or weakness of the teeth may respond to constitutional treatment. *Calc phos*, *calc fluor*, *mercurius*, *silica*, *staphisagria* and *thuja* types are among those most prone. See them in the remedy section, and consult the constitutional remedy finder for more suggestions. If a remedy is clearly indicated: that remedy potency 30, Regime F. Otherwise consult a homoeopath.

ULCERS, MOUTH

Ulcers, with increased salivation, metallic taste in the mouth, perhaps bad breath: *mercurius 30*, Regime A1.

Very painful, like sharp splinters; especially if ulcers are close to the salivary ducts; perhaps with angry mood: *nitric acid 30*, Regime A1.

Ulcers with signs of pus; pain made worse by cold things and relieved by warmth: *hepar sulph 30*, Regime A1.

If none of the above apply: *borax 30*, Regime A1.

Constitutional treatment

Recurrent or stubborn mouth ulcers need constitutional treatment, to which they usually respond well. Among the types most prone are *calc carb* (very common in plump children), *aurum*, *arsen alb*, *borax*, *lachesis*, *mercurius* and *nitric acid*. See them in the remedy section, and consult the constitutional remedy finder for more suggestions. If a remedy is well indicated: that remedy potency 30, Regime A1 during attacks, or potency 200 between them.

ULCERS, SKIN

Where the ulcer is clearly forming on a varicose vein; or with a tendency to slowly bleed dark red blood: *hamamelis 30*, Regime A.

Ulcer well-established, painful, discharging pus and fluid, perhaps smells rather offensive: *mercurius 30*, Regime A.

Ulcers discharging much pus; painful, and the pain is made much worse by pressure around the area and by cold; the patient generally chilly and perhaps in an irritable mood: *hepar sulph 30*, Regime A.

Ulcer with burning pains that are relieved by heat, in thin-built, anxious, chilly individuals: *arsen alb 30*, Regime A.

Ulcers where the area is distinctly blue or purple; worse or started on the left side; pains and the patient generally worse for heat: *lachesis 30*, Regime A.

Ulcers that develop slowly, not much pus or pain but very slow to heal;

in lightly-built, mild-tempered individuals: *silica 30*, Regime A.
Where poor circulation is clearly the root cause; alongside any of the above, or if none are indicated, to improve oxygenation to the area: *carbo veg 30*, Regime A. (If another remedy is also being taken, wait about an hour before having this one.)

Local application
As well as any of the above: *calendula mother tincture*, Regime N, or *calendula cream*, Regime M.

Individualised treatment

If none of the above is indicated or effective individualised treatment may help more. Apart from the above remedies, *calc carb*, *graphities*, *lycopodium*, *psorinum* and *pulsatilla* types are among those prone to this problem. If one is well indicated: that remedy potency 30, Regime A. Otherwise see a homoeopath.

ULCERS, STOMACH AND DUODENAL
(Also see Stomach Pain; Nausea and Vomiting)

Suspected or confirmed ulcer, gnawing pain comes on about two hours after eating; perhaps with desire to burp but difficulty doing so, or tendency to constipation; in irritable, chilly, individuals: *nux vomica 30*, Regime B1.

Suspected or confirmed ulcer; burning, acidic pain comes on during or just after eating, perhaps with nausea or vomiting; in chilly, anxious individuals: *arsen alb 30*, Regime B1.

Suspected or confirmed ulcer; gnawing pain comes on during or just after eating; with much flatulence passing downwards; pains tend to be worse on the right side; symptoms worse before an important event: *lycopodium 30*, Regime B1.

Suspected or confirmed ulcer; burning pains; much flatulence and burping; craving for salty and especially sugary foods, which aggravate the symptoms; in restless, warm-blooded individuals especially when worried about what is going to happen: *argent nit 30*, Regime B1.

If a stomach ulcer has been confirmed, this remedy has often helped repair the stomach lining, alone or in conjunction with other remedies: *ornithogalum mother tincture*, Regime E5.

If nothing else helps, while seeking advice: *hydrastis mother tincture*, Regime E5.

Individualised and constitutional treatment

Gastric ulcers respond best to constitutional treatment. In fact the suggestions above often develop from or into a constitutional state. Apart from them, other types prone to this problem include *anacardium*, *kali bich*, *phosphorus*, *psorinum*, *sepia* and *silica*. See them in the remedy section, and consult the constitutional remedy finder for more suggestions. If a remedy is well indicated: that remedy potency 30, Regime B1. In general it is advisable to see a homoeopath, as this condition generally responds well to accurate treatment, avoiding the need for more radical solutions later on.

VACCINATIONS

Bad reactions to vaccinations
First look up the symptoms of the reaction in the relevant section, such as fevers, sore throat, or whatever it is, and if a remedy is indicated, give it. Alongside that, or if nothing is indicated: *thuja 200*, Regime K.

Homoeopathic alternatives to vaccinations

Strictly speaking, there is no such thing. The two systems are based on completely different theories about the nature of health and disease. What many people have done is used nosodes (see p. 197) as a way of protecting themselves against particular conditions. No claims or guarantees about the efficacy of this method can be made. Anecdotal evidence is positive regarding its use for limited periods such as while travelling. It could not establish long-term immunity, in the way that conventional vaccinations are intended to do for childhood and other diseases.

Regime for nosodes while travelling or during periods of particular risk (several may be combined if necessary)
The nosode (e.g. malaria nosode, cholera nosode) 30, Regime F5 for trips of up two weeks, or Regime K1 for longer trips.

VAGINAL PROBLEMS
(Also see Female Reproductive System Problems; Sexual Problems)

Discharge, thrush
Around the period, or during pregnancy or menopause; white or yellow, perhaps burning, maybe profuse; in chilly women, and perhaps little girls; quick-tempered and tearful: *sepia 30*, Regime A.

Thick white or yellow discharge; perhaps before the period or in pregnancy, or in little girls; generally needs fresh air; placid or needy and tearful mood: *pulsatilla 30*, Regime A.

White discharge, perhaps causing soreness; perhaps before the period; with irritable, sensitive but reserved mood: *natrum mur 30*, Regime A.

Acrid, yellow discharge; in thin-built, chilly, anxious and fastidious individuals: *arsen alb 30*, Regime A.

Also see constitutional treatment below.

Dryness and pain
At menopause or with irritable, sensitive or resentful, but reserved mood; strong wish to be alone; perhaps also headaches or cystitis: *natrum mur 30*, Regime A.

Feeling emotionally put-upon and averse to being touched; craving to be left alone; perhaps with bearing-down pains, or backache: *sepia 30*, Regime A.

Also see constitutional treatment below.

Itching
During pregnancy or perhaps with or from leucorrhea: *sepia 30*, Regime A.

Worst before the period: *sulphur 30*, Regime B.

Worst after sex, or during or after the period: *natrum mur 30*, Regime B1.

Worse during urination: *mercurius 30*, Regime B1.

Also see constitutional treatment below.

Offensive discharges
Such conditions may have been diagnosed as a specific infection. For homoeopathic treatment, it is the actual symptoms experienced that are most important.

Smell like old cheese: *hepar sulph 30*, Regime A.

Fishy smell; with uncomfortably self-conscious state of mind: *thuja 200*, Regime C.

Fishy smell; with high sex-drive: *medorrhinum 200*, Regime C.

Also see constitutional treatment below.

Vaginismus

After emotional trauma: *ignatia 200*, Regime C.

In emotionally sensitive but unexpressive women: *natrum mur 200*, Regime C.

With shyness or anxiety about the partner's thoughts: *lycopodium 200*, Regime C.

With pain, cystitis or sexual frustration: *cantharis 30*, Regime B1.

Without obvious cause, nothing else is indicated: *mag phos 30*, Regime B1.

Constitutional treatment

If none of the suggestions above are appropriate or effective, constitutional treatment is needed, to which these conditions generally respond well.

Calc carb, *causticum*, *graphities*, *kali carb* and *silica* types are among those prone to vaginal discharges.

Lycopodium, *natrum mur*, *sepia* and *silica* types are prone to dryness.

Itching often affects *medorrhinum*, *natrum mur*, *nitric acid*, *sepia* and *thuja* types.

Natrum mur, *sepia* and *staphisagria* types are prone to vaginal pain. Also vulnerable are *argent nit*, *lycopodium*, *pulsatilla* and *thuja* individuals.

Sepia, *staphisagria* and *platina* are among the types that may also be prone to vaginismus.

Offensive discharges can affect *medorrhinum*, *sepia* and *thuja* individuals in particular.

Consider those remedies in the remedy section, and see the constitutional remedy finder for more suggestions. If a remedy is clearly indicated: that remedy potency 30, Regime A during episodes, or potency 200, Regime C between them. Otherwise consult a homoeopath.

VARICOSE VEINS

Recent varicose veins, after long periods of standing or perhaps during pregnancy or other times of change; patient intolerant of heat; rather placid or weepy state of mind: *pulsatilla 30*, Regime A.

Itchy or painful, worse standing, worse for heat, although the patient may be generally chilly: *sulphur 30*, Regime A.

Varicose veins with signs of ulceration (see Ulcers, Skin) especially if worse on left side: *lachesis 30*, Regime A.

None of the above is clearly indicated: *hamamelis 30*, Regime A.

Constitutional treatment

Stubborn or recurrent cases need constitutional treatment. Among the types prone to the problem are *arsen alb*, *calc carb*, *lachesis*, *lycopodium*, *pulsatilla* and *sulphur*. See them in the remedy section, and consult the constitutional remedy finder for more suggestions. If one is well indicated: that remedy potency 30, Regime A. Otherwise consult a homoeopath.

VERRUCAE

Thuja mother tincture, Regime N1, and *thuja 30*, Regime F.

VERTIGO, GIDDINESS, LABYRINTHITIS

Marked dizziness during an acute illness, especially fevers or headaches and during the early stages; better sitting up: *belladonna 30*, Regime B1.

Marked dizziness during an acute illness; very much worse rising or any movement of the head; irritable mood: *bryonia 30*, Regime B1.

Vertigo after a binge, heavy drinking, or period of overindulgence: *nux vomica 30*, Regime A.

Attacks of vertigo, perhaps after long periods of strain, or from disturbed sleep; perhaps diagnosed labyrinthitis: *cocculus 30*, Regime B1.

Attacks of vertigo, perhaps with nausea, together or alternating with noises in the ear; perhaps diagnosed Ménière's disease: *china sulph 30*, Regime B1.

Recurrent giddiness, worse looking up or down and out walking; in lightly-built, affectionate and impressionable individuals: *phosphorus 200*, Regime C.

Dizziness, particularly on turning the head, as when looking to cross the road; particularly in heavily-built and older people: *calc carb 200*, Regime C.

Constitutional treatment

If none of the above is effective, constitutional treatment is needed. This is particularly so in cases of diagnosed Ménière's or labyrinthitis, even if the remedies above help a little in the short term.

Argent nit, calc carb, cocculus, lycopodium, natrum mur, pulsatilla and *phosphorus* types are among those most prone to this sort of problem. See them in the remedy section, and consult the constitutional remedy finder for more suggestions. If a remedy is well indicated: that remedy potency 30, Regime B1 during attacks, or potency 200, Regime C between them. Otherwise see a homoeopath.

VOICE, LOST, HOARSE, LARYNGITIS
(Also see Throat; Coughs)

Voice hoarse or completely lost, perhaps during a cough or cold, or from over-use, symptoms worse for talking, laughing or breathing in; larynx painfully sore; generally affectionate mood or disposition: *phosphorus 30*, Regime B1.

Voice hoarse or completely lost, perhaps during a cough or cold, or from over-use; larynx feels weak or rigid; not particularly painful: *causticum 30*, Regime B1.

Voice hoarse, deep or completely lost, perhaps during a cough or cold or after being chilled; feeling very lethargic and cold but in need of fresh air: *carbo veg 30*, Regime B1.

Voice lost, from over-use, particularly singing; none of the above particularly applies: *arum tryph 30*, Regime B1.

Constitutional treatment

Stubborn or recurrent episodes need constitutional treatment to which they often respond well. *Phosphorus* and *causticum* types are very prone to the problem, but *carbo veg, hepar sulph, silica* and *sulphur* types can also be affected. Consider them in the remedy section, and see the constitutional remedy finder for more suggestions. If a remedy is well indicated: that remedy potency 30, Regime B1 during attacks, or potency 200, Regime C between them. Otherwise see a homoeopath.

NOTE: giving causticum and phosphorus. As mentioned in the remedy section, *phosphorus* and *causticum* are one of several pairs of incompatible remedies; if given in succession they can stimulate unpleasant aggravations of the symptoms. The two can be difficult to distinguish in cases of laryngitis. If one of them has been given and it is wished to try the other, first give one dose of *nux vomica* or *sulphur*, wait an hour, and then the other remedy can be administered safely.

WARTS

Specific remedy
Thuja mother tincture, Regime N1, and *thuja 30*, Regime F.

Constitutional treatment

Warts will sometimes respond to constitutional treatment. *Calc carb*, *causticum*, *lycopodium*, *medorrhinum*, *nitric acid* and *thuja* types are among those particularly prone. If any of them as described in the remedy section of this book fits well: that remedy potency 30, Regime F. Otherwise see a homoeopath.

WORMS

Itchy anus, patient driven to scratch the anus and perhaps to pick at the nose; very bad-tempered: *cina 30*, Regime A.
Itchy anus, without marked change of mood or nose-picking: *teucrium mar 30*, Regime A.
Worms, with colicky pains: *natrum phos 30*, Regime A.
If none of the above helps, or the patient suffers frequently repeated episodes: *carcinosin 200*, Regime C.

WRIST PROBLEMS

Repetitive strain injury
Pain and weakness of the wrist and fingers; much stiffness, unable to

exert pressure or hold things properly, sore pains, worse for cold and damp; where tendons and ligaments seem to be most affected: *ruta 30*, Regime F2.

Pains in fingers or shooting pains going up the arm; worse for cold, damp and movement; perhaps with pins and needles or tingling in the fingers; where nerves seem to be most affected: *hypericum 30*, Regime F2.

Wrist and hand go into painful spasm after using them, for example after gardening or sport, or as in writer's cramp; perhaps with or alternating with pins and needles or numbness; better for massage, warmth and rest: *mag phos 30*, Regime B1.

Pain and stiffness, worse when still and when first moving, better for warmth and continued movement; perhaps pins and needles: *rhus tox 30*, Regime F2.

Sore, bruised pain, worse for exertion and touch, better for warmth and rest: *arnica 30*, Regime F2.

Cramps or spasms, burning pains, perhaps pins and needles; general tiredness of body and mind; symptoms worse for heat and better cool, also better for bandaging: *picric acid 30*, Regime F2.

Weakness and progressive loss of movement in the wrists and hands, with a feeling as if the tendons were shortening; perhaps with pins and needles of the fingers: *causticum 30*, Regime F2.

Unable to move the wrist and parts of the hand in certain positions, pain in the parts that cannot be moved: *plumbum 30*, Regime F2.

Carpal tunnel syndrome
Pain or weakness diagnosed as carpal tunnel syndrome: see the suggestions for repetitive strain injury, above.

If adhesions, calcification or contraction of ligaments or tendons are contributing to carpal tunnel syndrome: *calc fluor 12*, Regime F6 (may be taken alongside one of the remedies above).

Constitutional and individualised treatment

If none of the above is appropriate or effective, constitutional treatment for overall strength and resilience might help. *Causticum*, *calc carb*, *graphities*, *lycopodium* and *phosphoric acid* are among the types most prone to this sort of problem. Consider them in the remedy section, and if one is well indicated: that remedy potency 30, Regime F2. Otherwise see a homoeopath.

Remedies A–Z

ACONITE, acon

Remedy source: plant—monkshood (*Aconitum napellus*).

Main uses

Aconite is used mainly as a quick-acting remedy for high temperatures and for the early stages of infectious conditions. It is also the greatest of remedies for the short- and long-term effects of intense fear or shock.

Fevers, colds and other acute conditions
If a condition has just come on and few symptoms are showing so far, aconite is very likely to be the best remedy. (The other main possibilities are belladonna and ferrum phos). It is frequently the first remedy needed during infectious childhood diseases, often before a diagnosis is possible and there is just a high temperature and obvious discomfort. Aconite conditions come on suddenly, often in the middle of the night, and the patient is anxious and restless. There may be high fever, little sweat, much thirst and a dry cough.

Aconite is also likely to be needed after someone has had a severe chill. The problem may come on straight away or later in the night after the exposure occurred. Then suddenly the patient wakes with earache or other symptoms.

Fear
Aconite is indicated when a person is simply terrified—for example, about flying or performing, or perhaps appearing in court. The person is very restless with the fear, or in extreme cases may be paralysed. The fear is not about anything complex or mysterious: it is like the fear of imminent death, with or without a rational basis.

The effects of fear

Any condition after severe fright or shock, however long ago the events happened, may need aconite. Even if other remedies are required later, aconite is sometimes the only one that can resolve the impact of such fear. Simple terror, rational or otherwise, like the fear of death, indicates aconite.

AGARICUS MUSCARIUS, agaricus, agar

Remedy source: fungus—fly agaric, bug agaric.

Main uses

This is quite an unusual remedy. It is useful in certain specific conditions, and there are also some psychological characteristics although these do not yet really add up to a well-understood constitutional type.

Specific conditions

Chilblains. Intense burning and itching, made worse by cold.

Nervous conditions. All sorts of neurological problems with twitching, spasms and even convulsions. Particularly of the eyelids, but possibly of any muscle group.

Mental and constitutional characteristics

Among the mental symptoms so far observed is a remarkable fearlessness, like children who go to complete strangers, or who climb and explore any place with apparently no sense of danger at all. Agaricus may be used in hyperactivity or slow development in children with this fearlessness. Adult cases of agaricus usually include many delusions, as if intoxicated. The person talks a great deal, jumping wildly from one subject to another. A marked fear of disease, in particular cancer, has been noted.

At least the beginnings of the typical nervous disorders are usually present where agaricus is prescribed. Symptoms begin with involuntary twitchings of single parts such as the eyelids. In the later stages appear uncontrollable or very exaggerated movements; perhaps the whole head moves and all the neck and shoulder muscles are involved in the simplest acts of speech.

Agaricus patients are usually very chilly and sensitive to cold. Sex may make the symptoms worse.

AGNUS CASTUS, agnus

Remedy source: plant—the chaste tree.

Main uses

The main homoeopathic use of this plant is in cases of lost or reduced sexual powers and desire, the opposite of its main herbal or naturopathic role. It is also sometimes given for fluid imbalances during times of hormonal change. This is in line with its herbal use.

AILANTHUS GLANDULOSA, ailanthus, ail

Remedy source: plant—ailanthus, tree of heaven.

Main uses

This is not a commonly used remedy, being given mostly during low-grade, perhaps protracted, feverish conditions.

Characteristics
The patient is hopelessly tired and prostrated, and the state of mind is one of dull confusion.

Physically, the glands of the face and neck are swollen and sore to touch. Dry, sore throat, dark red or even bluish, better for hot drinks. Perhaps coughing up small amounts of infected mucus. A sensation like an electric current running through the body is very characteristic.

The patient has been too ill, too long for gelsemium to work any more. At the same time, the system seems to be full of toxins as in blood-poisoning or a bad flu, but the symptoms are less vivid than those of other remedies such as baptisia, and aching in the limbs and back is not prominent. The condition just seems to stay the same without getting better or worse. From these features ailanthus has attained some notoriety as a specific for glandular fever and similar conditions.

ALLIUM CEPA, allium, all-c

Remedy source: plant—the red onion.

Main uses

Allium is quite widely used, mostly as a quick-acting remedy for colds and allergic conditions. It is indicated during colds and allergic reactions when the eyes and nose are streaming. The discharge from the eyes is bland, the runny nose makes the upper lip sore. There is violent sneezing. The left eye and nostril are most affected. Symptoms are better outside.

ALUMINA, alum

Remedy source: aluminium oxide.

Main uses

Alumina is used mostly as a specific remedy for constipation and problems of the nervous system. There is also a constitutional type, although it is not one that is particularly common or well described.

Constipation
Constipation when there is no urge to go (which is the same as opium and bryonia, and the opposite of nux vomica), but if and when the individual can pass a stool, it is still soft (unlike opium and bryonia where the stool is very hard). Alumina has been observed to work particularly well in old people with this kind of constipation, and in children who have been consuming artificial foods.

Nervous conditions
The features of aluminium poisoning have become well known through recent concern about cooking utensils. Homoeopathically alumina is used to treat conditions starting with poor memory and concentration, and progressing to numbness, paralysis and increasingly severe loss of nervous control.

The constitutional type

All the problems seem to go straight to the nervous system. At first the patient feels the need to hurry all the time, and is therefore restless and incapable of really enjoying anything. There is growing confusion about personal identity—for example, patients might say that in relationships they become strangely mixed up and lost in the identity of the other person, or that when they say something they are unsure if it was they who said it or someone else.

In this state of mind the world becomes a threatening place and the individual feels strong, irrational impulses to strike back at something or someone, impulses that may be triggered off by the sight of a knife, or of blood. Later there may be a tendency to the characteristic constipation or nervous problems. Concentration and memory degenerate so that any attempt to hurry such people along is unbearable. Gradually they develop physical numbness, paralysis and loss of control.

AMYL NITRATE, amyl-nit, amyl-n

Remedy source: the chemical.

When used, amyl nitrate is almost always used as a specific remedy for hot flushes, usually during the menopause, either alone or alongside constitutional remedies. There is sudden reddening of the face, followed by great heat and sometimes sweating. The person must have fresh air. The remedy may be used for sunstroke.

ANACARDIUM ORIENTALE, anacardium, anac

Remedy source: plant—the Indian marking nut.

Main uses

Anacardium is mostly used as a constitutional remedy. Apart from the mind it affects the stomach and skin, and very occasionally it is used as a specific remedy for conditions of those parts.

The constitutional type

Most symptoms are of the mind. The individual suffers an intense lack of self-confidence, a feeling that when the demands of daily life present themselves he will be unable either to cope or to evade them, so he dares not expose himself to anything and ceases to function at all. Or he thinks that everyone really feels this way, that fear is the rule of life, and he is driven to constantly prove himself. He becomes unfeeling, capable of cruelty, and driven to virulent profanity. The patient feels either of these states, or they may alternate or succeed one another. Then he feels himself pulled apart by wildly differing impulses, between refinement and diabolical urges.

The remedy may be given when just the first symptoms are present. These are lack of concentration and poor memory. Subsequently depression sets in. Personality disorders develop only in the most severe cases.

When they do, the root is psychological trauma, caused by either a particular event, or by long periods of being obliged to act in ways that go against one's own nature, such as the son under intense pressure to follow in his father's footsteps despite very different inclinations and aptitudes. A denial of personal space can trigger the anacardium condition, like the well-mannered citizen driven to homicidal rage by inconsiderate neighbours. (This makes anacardium an important remedy among contemporary city-dwellers, according to some homoeopaths). A common feature is the helplessness: the fury rises because inhibitions prevent effective confrontation with the source of torment.

On a physical level the symptoms involve the digestion, or intense irritation of the skin. Anacardium types are prone to all sorts of gastric troubles, from indigestion through ulceration to malignancy. Commonly the patient feels that something is stuck, like a plug, somewhere in the upper gastro-intestinal tract. A very characteristic feature is that the symptoms are relieved by eating, and this is true of mental states as well. The skin symptoms are eruptions like blisters that itch or burn, relieved by heat.

ANTIMONIUM CRUDUM, antim crud, ant-c

Remedy source: the element antimony.

Main uses

This remedy is mostly used during acute illnesses, and there is a constitutional type as well.

The constitutional type

Psychologically these individuals are touchy: they are easily irritated, and at the same time quickly moved to tears by sentimental feelings.

If they make a suggestion or invitation to a member of their family or a friend who does not respond in an entirely enthusiastic and willing manner, antim crud individuals sense their reserve immediately and do not disguise their discontent. Equally, displays of affection move them very much. Younger antim crud individuals are prone to episodes of lovesickness, more ridiculous than touching to others, however painful to themselves. Often they are sincerely sensitive people, who have been made to think that one must express one's feelings in obvious ways, or be ignored.

Physically, most of the effects are on the stomach and metabolism or skin. Antim crud types are heavily built and generally warm-blooded, with the characteristic tendency to irritability alternating with sentimentality or emotional dramatism. Small children who need this remedy are simply very bad-tempered and particularly intolerant of being touched or looked at. These types are prone to problems with the nails, which thicken and crack.

Short-term conditions

Stomach problems. Indigestion from rich food, especially pastry. The patient is sensitive to heat and cold but especially intolerant of stuffiness, and irritable. A strong indication for antim crud is a thick, white coating on the tongue. If the tongue is clean, this remedy is very unlikely to help.

Skin problems. The patient is irritable, and in particular does not want to be looked at. Often there is nausea or other stomach problems with the skin troubles. This is the main remedy for straightforward cases of impetigo if nothing else is indicated.

ANTIMONIUM TARTARICUM, antim tart, ant-t

Remedy source: tartar emetic.

Main uses

Antim tart is very widely used as a specific remedy for coughs. No constitutional type has been identified.

Characteristics
Antim tart is mostly used during acute illnesses when the main symptom is a cough that is loose and rattly but produces little actual expectoration.

Another important indication is that the patient is weak and tired and, in particular, very sleepy. The patient is often hot and intolerant of warmth.

It is one of the most widely used remedies for acute loose coughs in children, and both acute and ongoing coughs of the elderly. It may be that the circulation to the lungs is at fault. Often just the loose cough is enough for antim tart to be prescribed successfully, and if the weakness, warmth and sleepiness are also present it can be given with confidence.

APIS MELLIFICA, apis mel, apis

Remedy source: the honey bee.

Main uses

Apis is quite widely used as an acute remedy for allergic reactions, stings and skin afflictions, and sometimes as a constitutional type.

Acute symptoms
Bearing in mind that the remedy is made from a whole bee, the acute symptoms of this remedy are quite easy to remember. Symptoms often resemble a histamine reaction—hence, allergic reactions, stings, eruptions or swellings which contain lots of fluid, like swollen bags or blisters, and the area is hot to the touch, stinging or itchy, bright or shiny red, made worse by heat and relieved by cold. A helpful indication is that the patient has surprisingly little or no thirst.

Apis can also help with water retention, where the area is not so hot and red and just a lot of fluid is being retained in certain parts. This is usually a short-term measure, not a real cure, in cases which come on occasionally in situations like intense heat or around the menstrual period.

Constitutional characteristics

Again the features of the bee give a lot of useful reminders. Mentally, apis individuals are busy. If there is nothing useful to do, they find something else, and never seem to rest. In their haste and agitation they are awkward, clumsy people who drop things and bang into objects. They dislike being disturbed or distracted from their work and often react with stinging comments. They generally talk a lot, not necessarily loudly, but more or less continuously and to little purpose. They are often highly sexed. They are jealous in a territorial way, and the symptoms may be brought on by jealousy and anger.

Physical characteristics
Apis types are almost always hot people who do not tolerate heat, often again with the odd thistlessness. They are prone to the kind of swellings and allergic reactions seen in the acute situations, and there may be problems of the urinary and reproductive systems, particularly in women. If one side is affected, it is usually the right. Predominantly left-sided symptoms point strongly against apis (and towards lachesis, which resembles apis in many ways).

ARGENTUM NITRICUM, argent nit, arg nit
Remedy source: silver nitrate.

Main uses

Mostly a constitutional remedy. Sometimes used specifically for nerves before events.

The constitutional type

This remedy is for disturbed, agitated conditions of the mind and nerves. Individuals are subject to disordered sense-perceptions: objects seem to move or distances are distorted. Inwardly, they experience peculiar and persistent suggestions to do strange things, like jump from high places, and generally to expect the orderly condition of the world to dissolve into anarchy. Whatever solution to a problem is suggested, their mind presents some weird objection, and however safe things appear they expect a fluke catastrophe.

The symptoms begin with restlessness, for no apparent reason. Then strong phobias develop, of almost any kind. Individuals are particularly badly affected by anxiety about any forthcoming event, even something apparently trivial. The anticipatory anxiety grows out of all proportion, making them restless, forgetful and confused. This is perhaps the most characteristic feature of the argent nit personality.

The mind predominates over the emotions. Almost all the inner energy is being used by the brain and nerves. They can appear most quick-witted and articulate.

There are some physical features that have to be present for argent nit to be prescribed with confidence and which often draw the homoeopath's attention to this remedy while the mental symptoms are only first appearing. The individual is almost always hot—these types go around in T-shirts in mid-winter. They crave sugary foods, and their digestion is affected. Most of all they get severe flatulence and bloating, or diarrhoea, or both, all aggravated by the sugar. Oddly, the pains are made better by strong pressure to the affected part.

Specific uses
Because argent nit types suffer so badly with nerves before events, the remedy is often suggested for this problem. It will only do much good if other symptoms of the argent nit personality are present, such as the restlessness, desire for sweets, and flatulence. If so, the remedy will probably help a lot. If not it will do little good and better results are likely from aconite or gelsemium.

ARNICA MONTANA, arnica, arn

Remedy source: plant—leopard's bane.

Main uses

Arnica is perhaps the most widely used homoeopathic remedy of them all, justly celebrated for its power over the effects of injury. It protects against shock, stems the flow of bleeding, reduces pain to a considerable degree, and promptly initiates the process of healing to all tissues. Given in high potencies it can resolve the residual effects of injuries and traumas, physical and psychological, years or even decades after the event.

Characteristics
After any accident or injury arnica may be given to good effect before any other action is taken, apart from summoning necessary medical aid. But like all remedies it has its characteristic symptoms in the absence of which its effects will be limited. Its real sphere of action is where trauma has caused 'extravasion'—that is blood or other bodily fluids have been forced out of their proper channels. Most often this means bruising, where blood is expelled from the capillaries, but extravasion of the fluid accommodating nerves and other tissues can equally be restored by arnica.

Subjectively the patient is sore and tender, and is usually anxious to avoid any more contact with the affected part. Of course the child cries out for comfort, but in some cases the instinct to protect the injury from further agitation leads even a seriously injured person to insist that little is wrong and no attention is needed.

Old injuries

Almost any pain or complaint that definitely began after trauma may be benefited by arnica. Where there is pain in a limb, soreness of the back, or even malfunction in an organ, which started after a blow or other injury, arnica should be considered. If the event was years ago, the highest potencies will be needed. In such cases arnica could be given in between other remedies.

Arnica is sometimes the remedy for long-standing psychological trauma such as shock, and particularly a true mental blow from which the mind has never fully recovered. In such cases one would expect to see the characteristic tenderness that instinctively avoids more touching on the sore point and perhaps thus denies the existence of a problem to be addressed; it is this that would point to arnica rather than another psychological trauma remedy such as ignatia.

Specific uses

Arnica can relieve some on-going physical pains such as rheumatism and sore backs. It will help in those cases where there are sore, bruised pains, made worse by touch. Throughout childbirth arnica is a great support, reducing discomfort and bleeding. The period of recovery after operations is dramatically reduced by arnica. Recently it has been observed to resolve or prevent the effects of jet-lag.

ARSENICUM ALBUM, arsen alb, ars

Remedy source: white arsenic.

Main uses

Arsenicum is very often used, both in short-term illnesses and as a constitutional type.

Short-term uses

Arsen alb is the first remedy for acute vomiting and diarrhoea. If nothing else is indicated or time is limited, this is usually the remedy to give first. It is also often indicated in mature colds and coughs.

The really characteristic symptoms of arsen alb are anxiety, restlessness, fussiness, and a real fear of being left alone. Usually one of these psychological features is apparent in even the most obvious cases of vomiting and diarrhoea from bad food, or in cases of chest infection.

On the physical level patients are chilly. They are also thirsty, but drink only small amounts at a time. If the cough is productive, the phlegm is white or frothy. Discharges, from the nose, eyes or anywhere else, are acrid and make the area sore.

The constitutional type

The constitutional type shares many of the acute symptoms. Arsen alb individuals are anxious, restless and conscientious. The anxiety drives them to constant activity. At work they pack their schedule, and they pursue leisure activities in the same spirit. Generally some part of their body is in constant motion, whatever they are doing.

What they worry about most is money and health. The fear of being alone is deep and intense. They like to surround themselves with experts, and expect them to know what is best. Their personal lives may resemble a network of support systems rather than human relationships.

Their most visible trait is fastidiousness. In dress, manners and the arrangement of their homes and work-spaces, everything has a place and is kept to it. They believe that there is a right way for things to be and that the deplorable tendency of others to allow them to be otherwise is the cause of most of the trouble in the world. Arsenicum types are critical and censorious in their attitudes to others, and they often feel their opinions are to be expressed for the good of all concerned, rather than repressed. Their fastidiousness finds expression even physically: the symptoms come on at regular times and intervals.

The negative traits of character have been emphasised above, but so long as they remain mentally well balanced they are constructive, interesting people, with a natural authority and refreshing frankness of manner.

Body type

Metabolically they are chilly people who do not tolerate the cold at all well. The pains they suffer, in the abdomen or chest, tend to be of a burning quality, and even these are relieved by heat and aggravated by cold. The only exception is in the region of the head, where cool air or applications may help. These types are vulnerable to problems with the digestion, bowels, breathing, and sometimes skin. They are usually thin-built.

ARSENICUM IODATUM, arsen iod, ars iod

Remedy source: iodide of arsenic.

This remedy is very similar in its action to arsen alb. It shares the anxious, restless, fastidious state of mind, and the burning pains and discharges. The one big difference is that in the case of arsen iod the individual is hot and symptoms are made worse by heat, unlike the arsen alb type which is chilly and much relieved by warmth. For this reason arsen iod is often given in situations like hay fever, some chest infections and skin conditions.

As well as heat the iodatum element sometimes produces a condition of overactivity, and some homoeopaths think of arsen iod as an important remedy for hyperactivity in children. It has also been effective in skin conditions, particularly psoriasis, sometimes because it is indicated but often as a last resort when nothing else has worked.

ARUM TRIPHYLLUM, arum triph, arum-t

Remedy source: plant—Indian turnip, Jack in the pulpit.

Main uses

Arum is used almost exclusively for soreness of the larynx and loss of voice or hoarseness from overuse. In speakers and singers, where there are no clear indications for one of the constitutional remedies most prone to larynx problems (causticum, phosphorus), arum triph is often pleasingly helpful.

It is occasionally used in skin problems, such as impetigo. The area is sore and raw, and the patient is driven to constantly pick at the area, perhaps causing it to bleed.

ASARUM EUROPAEUM, asarum, asar

Remedy source: plant—hazel wort, wild nath.

The constitutional type

This remedy is almost always used as a constitutional remedy. It is not a very common type.

Psychological and nervous features

A feature that is almost always present, and which usually leads the homoeopath to consider this remedy, is great sensitivity of hearing— particularly to noises like fingers being scraped, but also to high-pitched, penetrating or simply loud noises of any kind. Such noises cause not only discomfort to the ears but often physical pain in any part of the body.

The patient is sensitive on other levels. The emotions are affected in a certain way that makes them hard to express, leading to depression and apathy. A very characteristic symptom is a feeling like shivers caused by emotions. Instead of gladness or unhappiness in response to events, the individual experiences a sort of inner shudder, and is left uncomfortably wondering how to respond to others. These difficulties lead to an apparent aversion to giving and taking affection, in particular sexually, although this is due ultimately to an excess of emotional sensitivity rather than its absence.

Asarum types are usually cerebral individuals doing jobs that involve their minds and senses much more than their bodies. The tension they feel leads to a strong desire for alcohol or other sedative substances, and this desire and the effort of will needed to control it can become a major issue in their lives.

Physical features

On a physical level patients get aches and pains in the head and elsewhere which feel like something pressing outwards. As well as the sensitivity of hearing, they are prone to other ear problems, including tinnitus. They are chilly types.

AURUM METALLICUM, aurum met, aurum, aur

Remedy source: the element gold.

Main uses

Aurum is almost exclusively used as a constitutional remedy.

The constitutional characteristics

When this remedy is prescribed depression is almost always an important feature of the patient's condition. In advanced stages aurum types feel a hopeless, helpless, black depression. They think of death as a relief and seriously consider suicide. Even in less developed cases profound melancholy characterises the patients' outlook, although they may manage to present an effective face to the world.

The depth of sadness in the aurum personality can be difficult to perceive, because another feature of the type is a strong sense of duty and responsibility. Aurum types are industrious and work with integrity. Their sense of right and wrong is acute. Characteristically they hate to be contradicted, and when they are their self-control may break down to reveal a furious irritability. They set high standards for themselves, and it is a sense of disappointment, in themselves or others or the universe as a whole, which is often at the bottom of their discontent.

Depression approaching suicide and a serious, responsible attitude are features shared with natrum sulphuricum. One difference is a certain emotional colour in aurum that is absent in natrum sulph. Aurum is aware of being sad. The individual conducts himself and may even give expression to his aching heart with some emotional force. Serious music is comforting to him. There is a spiritual element in his feelings, even if he does not know to whom or what it should be addressed. The biographies as well as the poetry of T.S. Eliot display many aurum characteristics. The natrum sulph individual, on the other hand, perceives the world with complete dispassion.

Physical symptoms
If there are physical symptoms in an aurum case they are usually in the bones, or the heart, or the testes or ovaries, particularly on the right side. Congenital defects also point towards a group of remedies that includes aurum. So too does a history in the family of self-destructiveness in some form, such as suicide or alcoholism.

One love aurum types sometimes indulge is the sun. To lie exposed under the golden solar rays for long periods brings relief to the aurum individual. This is the opposite of natrum mur, and can be a way of distinguishing between these two sad, sensitive, personality types.

BAPTISIA TINCTORIA, baptisia, bapt

Remedy source: plant—wild indigo.

Main uses

No constitutional type has been suggested. The most common use of baptisia is in acute feverish diseases, cases of influenza or gastric upsets, or in generalised septic states like food poisoning and even typhoid.

Characteristics
Symptoms are quite severe. The patient is very weak and tired, but the aching in the back and limbs is intense and the body feels sore, forcing him to move around restlessly. Most characteristic is a mental state of bewilderment and confusion: the patient is unsure of where he is, or of his control over his own body which seems to be 'in bits' around the bed. He is very nauseous, and the throat is deep red, even bluish. There are signs of sepsis like smelly discharges and breath.

Baptisia is a very useful remedy for travellers to new places to have with them. Potency 200 is good.

BARYTA CARBONICUM, baryta carb, bar-c

Remedy source: barium carbonate.

Main uses

Baryta carb is widely used as a constitutional remedy, and sometimes specifically for conditions of the mind and throat.

Characteristics
The most important symptom of baryta carb is childishness. It is the most-used remedy for slow development in children, and for deterioration of the mental faculties in older people. There are no symptoms of mania or mental disturbance, just a failure to develop beyond a certain level, or a return to the helpless state of a child. For such children the remedy can produce wonderful results; sadly, elderly brains respond less readily.

Baryta carb infants tend to be plump. They may eat and sleep well, but do not develop in other areas. Whether or not a case of learning difficulties or special needs has been diagnosed, they are slow to walk and talk, and perform the same simple actions repeatedly. They are rarely aggressive or destructive but seem to have little focus or interest in what is around them. The parents offer all the stimulation and support they can, but it makes little impression. Sometimes the child is very averse to being left alone, and cries loudly if left alone in a room.

Older baryta carb children or adults show different degrees of the same tendencies. Typically the personality remains unformed. They suffer a debilitating lack of confidence, difficulty in making decisions, and a reluctance to take on responsibilities or challenges to a degree that severely inhibits their lives. Individuals are distressed by the presence of strangers and hide behind the familiar. They can only respond to admonishment with nervous laughter. Frequently the body type is plump and rather childlike, in particular the genitals are prone to underdevelopment.

In exceptional cases such people are apparently well-developed with a keen mind and active life. But they are limited by severe lack of confidence and perhaps a concentration on one narrow interest to the exclusion of all else. A history of chronic tonsillitis and the childlike body type would also indicate baryta carb. In cases strongly characterised by such traits baryta carb may be needed at some point during treatment.

Specific uses
Apart from the almost routine use of this remedy noted above for juvenile underdevelopment and mental deterioration of the elderly, this remedy has been used effectively in cases of chronic tonsillitis, where none of the other symptoms are present but no other remedies are indicated or effective.

BARYTA MURIATICUM, baryta mur, bar-m

Remedy source: barium chloride.

Main uses

See baryta carb. Where a certain sexual promiscuity is present in cases that otherwise resemble the mental symptoms of baryta carb, a homoeopath may select baryta mur.

It has also been particularly effective in cases of chronic or recurrent tonsillitis with great swelling and sometimes suppuration, which linger after colds, particularly when the weather changes in spring or autumn.

BELLADONNA, bell

Remedy source: plant—deadly nightshade.

Main uses

This is one of the most widely used homoeopathic remedies, particularly in acute, feverish conditions. There are also some well-known mental symptoms, but they are more likely to appear as a short-term disorder involving the mind than as a constitutional type.

Fevers and inflammations
Belladonna is very likely to be indicated in the first stages of fevers, colds and inflammations where other symptoms have not fully developed. The patient is hot and red, the skin is often still dry rather than sweaty, and it is the sort of heat like a radiator that can be felt through bedclothes or across the room. Individual parts of the body that are affected are also bright red, such as ears and throat.

The pains are throbbing. The eyes are staring and pupils dilated, and strong light is painful. The patient often feels rather dizzy and, in severe cases, is delirious. Everything feels better sitting propped up rather than lying flat. Earaches, headaches and sore throats are usually worse on the right side. Symptoms often come on or get worse at around 3 p.m. The patient is very sensitive: apart from the photophobia, sudden external movements (such as someone jarring the bed) are very aggravating and there is sensitivity to draughts. The patient is very thirsty, and often asks for drinks with a sour taste, like lemon crushes or even beer. He may feel better for small quantities of light food.

If a condition is still in the early stages, has come on suddenly and this sort of full-blooded heat characterises the situation, belladonna is very likely to be the remedy. It is often the first remedy for childhood fevers where the only symptoms are heat and discomfort. At this point it often has to be distinguished from aconite, which is more acutely anxious and restless, and ferrum phos, where the symptoms are less intense and come on more slowly.

Other conditions
Belladonna can be indicated in other conditions that come on suddenly accompanied by the full-blooded heat—for example; sunstroke and headaches from the sun, right-sided throbbing headaches, right-sided mastitis, acute attacks of high blood pressure, and any such symptoms brought on by a sudden change of temperature or with hormonal changes or strong emotions.

Mental symptoms
Belladonna is indicated in some cases of mental disturbance approaching mania. Here it has to be distinguished from remedies like stramonium and hyoscyamus. With belladonna, the delirium characteristic of the feverish state recurs as vivid delusions. The patient becomes wildly bad-tempered, striking out and spitting, and the mania seems to increase his strength. The mania includes fears, most typically of big, black dogs. The excessive sensitivity is present, to light, noise and touch. Belladonna is most likely to help individuals who are generally happy and well balanced, but become severely disturbed when ill.

BELLIS PERENNIS, bellis per, bellis

Remedy source: plant—the daisy.

Main uses

Bellis is generally used as an acute remedy for certain kinds of injury. It seems to work mostly on the blood supply to muscles, placing it close to rhus tox and particularly arnica, and making it an important remedy for the effects of injuries and strains in those who do much physical work, in the elderly, and also in pregnancy.

Strains
Back and limbs sore and aching, from long periods of heavy work such as the stiff backs of labourers and regular gardeners, rather than a single act of over-lifting (which is likely to respond best to rhus tox). Pain and stiffness of the limbs and pelvis during pregnancy. Symptoms better for moving and being rubbed. Anything that improves the blood supply to the area is comforting.

Incisions

Deep wounds or surgical incisions, such as to the abdomen. After abdominal surgery bellis can help much to promote healing and minimise discomfort, perhaps taken alongside arnica or staphisagria.

Breasts

After a blow or injury to the breast, if arnica or phytolacca do not help much and discomfort lasts a long time, and particularly if the area becomes inflamed and hard.

BERBERIS AQUIFOLIUM, berb-a

Remedy source: plant—Oregon grape, mahonia.

Very little is known about this remedy except as a specific treatment for various skin conditions. Cases of acne and psoriasis have been known to respond well to it, where no other remedies were effective or indicated.

BERBERIS VULGARIS, berberis, berb

Remedy source: plant—barberry.

Main uses

This remedy is used mostly during acute illnesses centred on the kidneys, or sometimes alongside other remedies, in order to strengthen the kidneys. It also has some action on the liver.

Characteristics

It is often given in those cases where the kidneys are clearly involved, as indicated by pain in the region, where there are few other symptoms.

But berberis does have characteristic symptoms of its own. Most typical are pains that radiate, from and around the kidneys. And with berberis it is most often the left side that is affected.

It is one of the most important remedies for renal colic on the left side, or for cystitis, with pain in the region of the kidneys. It is indicated for disorders of the liver and gall bladder, with the typical pains radiating around the region, or alongside urinary problems.

Berberis is one of those remedies that is often given in very low potencies, even mother tincture.

BORAX, bor

Remedy source: a compound of boracic acid and sodium, widely used in Hahnemann's time.

Main uses

This remedy is used mostly for a few specific conditions, and the outline of the constitutional type has been described.

Specific uses

In cases of acute and occasional mouth ulcers with few other symptoms, borax is often surprisingly helpful. Another marked feature of the remedy is thick, creamy deposits, such as on the tongue or from the vagina, leading to its frequent use in thrush. The state of mind is generally mild and accommodating (unlike mercurius, the other main specific remedy for ulcers), and the individual is chilly and sensitive to cold (the opposite of pulsatilla, which has lots of thick discharges).

Constitutional features

Among the confirmed features of the borax type are delicate and oversensitive nerves. Such people are easily startled, and are particularly sensitive to loud, sudden noises. Firework celebrations are a nightmare for them. A very characteristic feature is a fear of downward motion, which can take many forms: children cry out and cling on when put down, and adults have literal fears or dreams of falling, such as in aircraft or escalators, and more subtle anxieties about their material security. If this symptom is a marked feature of the case, borax should be considered carefully. If it is missing, borax is unlikely to act deeply, if at all.

Borax people are generally chilly, slightly-built types. They frequently suffer from mouth ulcers, oral thrush, profuse vaginal discharges, headaches and skin problems such as dryness and herpetic eruptions, and eruptions around the eyes. Borax is often indicated for problems of nursing mothers and infants, and a particular symptom is pain in the opposite breast while feeding.

Sometimes the remedy is given specifically for fear of loud noises—for example, to pets on the nights of regular firework celebrations. In fact, unless the constitutional traits are present it will do little good in such circumstances, and a remedy like aconite would be more helpful.

BRYONIA ALBA, bryonia, bry

Remedy source: plant—white bryony, wild hops.

Main uses

This is a very widely used homoeopathic remedy, particularly during short-term conditions, although the constitutional type is quite well known as well.

Acute symptoms

Overwhelmingly, the most important characteristic of bryonia is that the symptoms are made worse by movement. It could be the pain of an injury or in tissues anywhere during an acute disease, but the condition is immediately and severely made worse by movement, and equally relieved by keeping completely still and quiet. This makes bryonia one of the most useful remedies for chest and throat infections with pain aggravated by coughing or any other movement. Also for headaches and migraines, as well as injuries or inflammations anywhere with that pattern. One thing to bear in mind is that the aggravation from movement is such that strong, constant pressure is comforting if it keeps the affected part still.

Related to the aggravation from movement is a very marked general dryness; of the throat, skin and any mucous membranes. This makes the individual thirsty for long drinks at long intervals. The fever or inflammation is often high or intense, causing a desire for cool air or drinks.

Mentally, too, the patient is dry and touchy and very irritable indeed, just wanting to be left alone and in peace. An odd and very characteristic outcome of the dryness is that despite being apparently really ill, the patient thinks and talks of work or the responsibilities he must attend to.

Constitutional symptoms

The dryness and aggravation from disturbance is also evident in the bryonia personality type. These individuals are constantly concerned with their work and worldly duties which might be quite laudable and constructive, but they are focused upon them to the exclusion of life's lighter, and deeper, aspects. As a cause or consequence of these habits of mind, deep anxiety arises about material security, described in the textbooks as fear of poverty.

These sensitivities and anxieties make bryonia people very irritable, possibly really nasty in fact, like nux vomica and hepar sulph. Just as in the acute symptoms the patient is worse for movement and better for hard pressure, so on the general mental level the individual resents disturbance and change, but at the same time feels compelled to take on a heavy workload and lots of responsibility.

Bryonia types are generally warm-blooded and aggravated by heat, as in the acute symptoms. They are prone to symptoms of the mind, head, chest and mucous membranes.

CALCAREA CARBONICA, calc carb, calc

Remedy source: mineral—chalky layer of the oyster shell.

Main uses

One of the most widely used homoeopathic remedies of them all, almost always prescribed on the basis of constitutional characteristics.

Psychological characteristics

The calc carb mind does not learn very fast, but retains what it has grasped. Individuals may be aware of being slow, and are rather afraid and irritated by things and people that move quickly. A well-known feature of the type is a sense of being confused, and a fear that others will notice this and take advantage. Being rushed is very disagreeable to them, and they generally refuse to allow it to happen. This can appear as stubbornness for its own sake. They are prone to anxieties and phobias, particularly about small fast-moving animals such as mice and insects.

Calc carb types may be quite philosophical, including the children. The sulphur child constantly asks 'why?' and pulls things to pieces, but calc carb children sit and reflect on the fundamentally inscrutable and unchangeable nature of things. They are sensitive individuals, affected particularly by sad news, even about people they do not know at all. Gentle people who cannot bear to hear of cruelties or watch the television news are very often calc carb types.

Calcium is an essential component in the formation of all higher life forms. A deficiency of it produces a limp, unformed condition; too much leads to heaviness and lack of adaptability. Calc carb is applied homoeopathically right across this vast spectrum of potential imbalances.

Physical features
Most calc carbs are on the plump side, with pale, soft flesh. They sweat easily, particularly on the head, but they feel the cold. Their taste is for predominantly bland, carbohydrate-orientated foods, and they have a particular liking for eggs and sweets, but milk disagrees with them. They are prone to colds which go on to the chest and clear up only slowly. Their backs and limbs tend to rheumatic conditions. Calc carb types are very prone to constipation—in fact passing stools only every second or third day becomes the norm and is not a problem. The faces of older calc carb types are often covered in deep wrinkles (which create an attractive, lived-in, characterful effect, not the pained frown-lines of lycopodium).

The calc carb child
The child of this type is plumply built, with pale, soft flesh, a large head and round abdomen. He tends to sweat, especially on the head, goes for rather bland foods and has many troubles with tooth development. He learns slowly but steadily and is rather self-conscious among children who move and think more quickly; this makes him oddly stubborn sometimes, but generally he is patient and even-tempered.

Specific uses
Calc carb could be indicated in relatively short-term conditions such as fevers or disturbances of the digestion, where there are strong calc carb symptoms such as the food desires. Calc carb children often require belladonna during acute episodes like fevers. The aches and pains of older calc carb individuals often respond best to rhus tox during flare-ups.

CALCAREA FLUORIDE, calc fluor, calc-f

Remedy source: the mineral compound.

Main uses

This remedy has specific applications relating mostly to bones and connective tissue, and the skeleton of a constitutional type has been identified.

Specific uses

Calcium fluoride is an important constituent of body parts such as the surface of bones, the enamel of teeth, in elastic fibres and in the cells of the skin. The homoeopathic remedy is used specifically in conditions where the problem arises from a general excess of this substance, such as bony growths, calcifications, and adhesions or loss of elasticity. In such situations, *calc fluor 6X* Regime F2 would be appropriate.

Constitutional features

The excessive rigidity characteristic of the remedy on a physical level manifests itself in the calc fluor mind as a preoccupation with fear of material loss, of poverty.

The body type of calc fluor individuals tends towards hypermobility and exaggerated flexibility of joints—that is, they lack the structure that appears to excess in the acute applications of the remedy. They are generally chilly types, aggravated by changes in weather. The pains in the back and joints have a pattern similar to that of rhus tox: pain on first motion, relieved by sustained movement, like a rusty hinge.

Apart from bone trouble they are prone to other chronic conditions arising from exertion, as in athletes and dancers. They also suffer weakness of teeth, cramps, cataracts and thyroid troubles.

CALCAREA PHOSPHORICUM, calc phos, calc-p

Remedy source: calcium phosphate.

Specific uses

Calc phos is often used for problems with the bones, and also for teeth and skin. It can be given after fractures to help bones heal, and in cases of general bone weakness, either in children or older people suffering osteoporosis. Calc phos can be prescribed for children who are teething, perhaps between or alongside other remedies for pain. It is also sometimes given for some chest infections, or more likely for a tendency to get them.

Constitutional characteristics

There is also a constitutional calc phos type. Such people are prone to problems with bones, skin, breathing, and sometimes headaches. It is one of the most important remedies for children who are not developing well. On a physical level they are small, thin-boned, thin-chested and prone to chest complaints, and the skin is dry and rough. They may be slow to learn to walk. Their difficulties with assimilation and development are typified by intolerance of milk, even that of their mothers.

They are discontented and restless individuals. In adults this often turns into a desire for constant travelling, while the calc phos child is constantly bored. The condition can be brought on in children and young adults through sustained over exertion, particularly mental work. This leads to mental apathy and headaches. Regarding food they love smoked things. They are generally chilly types, who hate draughts.

It is signs of generally poor assimilation and development, together with some of these well-known characteristics, that often draw a homoeopath's attention to the need for calc phos in a case. Unlike the calc carb and phosphorus types, a real understanding of the pattern and dynamics underlying these bits of data about calc phos is surprisingly undeveloped, rather like the conditions it is used to treat.

CALCAREA SULPHURICUM, calc sulph, calc-s

Remedy source: calcium sulphate, gypsum, plaster of Paris.

This remedy is not often used, surprisingly, given that other compounds of the two elements are among the most widely employed of all. When given, it is usually as a constitutional remedy, but almost always largely on the basis of one very characteristic symptom. This is a tendency to profuse or repeated pus-like discharges, which are thick and yellow, and which discharge easily. If this symptom is present, the homoeopath's attention is drawn to consider calc sulph carefully, and rarely otherwise. Then if the area is not so acutely inflamed and painful as expected in cases of hepar sulph and mercurius, and if the discharge flows easily, unlike situations requiring silica, calc sulph is further indicated.

If the patient is a heavily-built and warm-blooded person, and warmth tends to aggravate the symptoms, this too points to calc sulph. In some cases jealousy and a feeling that others do not appreciate his worth characterise the calc sulph mind, and if these features are present the remedy may be prescribed with particular confidence.

CALENDULA OFFICINALIS, calendula, cal

Remedy source: plant—pot marigold.

Calendula is very widely used as a local application for its antiseptic qualities and ability to promote the swift growth of new tissues after cuts and abrasions.

Whether it is applied neat as a tincture, diluted in water, in creams, gels or ointments, depends entirely on the suitability of the vehicle for the conditions of the tissues to which it is to be applied. It can be used on any parts. Cut and denuded flesh, cracked nipples, sore gums, fissures of the anus and skin eruptions, can also all safely benefit from it.

Less common but at least as effective is the use of calendula internally in potency. In the 30 or 200 potency given two or three times daily it facilitates and accelerates the development of healthy new tissue.

CAMPHORA, camphor, camph

Remedy source: camphor, gum of the camphor laurel tree.

Main uses

Camphor is mostly used as an acute remedy, in situations where the most prominent symptoms are coldness, weakness and shivering. There is also a constitutional type, which is not commonly prescribed but has some vivid symptoms.

Acute conditions
The beginning of a cold or other acute illness, where few symptoms have yet developed apart from a chill or general feeling of coldness, perhaps causing the individual to shiver. In more developed cases the patient needing camphor is weak to the point of collapse, with the characteristic chilliness and shivering, and at the same time an odd aversion to being covered up. In severe cases the lips and skin become blue. The patient is very cold to touch, but the internal coldness may alternate with a feeling of inner burning. The situation could be one of shock, from injury or cold. If someone has been badly chilled and is

feeling as if nothing can ever warm him up, camphor is likely to be the remedy. The main alternative is aconite, in cases where the patient is more energetic, restless and anxious.

It can be indicated in fevers and gastric disturbances, again with the coldness, weakness and aversion to covering. In the treatment of cholera, it has been effectively used by homoeopaths for centuries, and by practitioners of ayurvedic medicine perhaps for millennia.

Psychological and constitutional symptoms

Camphora has been used successfully as a constitutional remedy in cases characterised on all levels by coldness. The individual feels unwanted, uncared for and isolated. The perceived lack of sympathy disturbs the mind and feelings of hatred arise, bursting out sometimes in rage and destructiveness. A very characteristic symptom of camphor individuals is that pains are better when the patient thinks about them.

CANNABIS INDICA, cannabis ind, cann-i

Remedy source: plant—hashish.

Main uses

This remedy is a rather uncommon constitutional type, and is occasionally used as a specific medicine for some of the complaints to which the constitutional type is prone.

The constitutional type

Cannabis is not often indicated for people who regularly use the recreational drug, although it may be for their children.

Those who do benefit from it display, as one might expect, an extremely vivid imagination or dream-life, to the point that it profoundly colours their perception of the outer world as well, and sometimes they show a propensity for fantastic speculations and theorising. Among relatively healthy cannabis types a very characteristic feature is laughter. It is loud, inordinate, frequent, and usually infectious. Sometimes if the mind-set has become more fixed and disordered, there arises intense suspiciousness, approaching paranoia. If one or more of these traits are evident, a homoeopath will have to very carefully consider cannabis as the remedy; in their absence it is unlikely even to come up for consideration.

Typical problems

The most common conditions of the type arise from an exaggeration of their psychological traits—confusion, forgetfulness, exhaustion. The conditions are worse for stimulants and anything that further leaves them to their inner world, such as darkness.

Physically they are prone to problems with the genitals and urinary organs, including cystitis and spasms, and sometimes painful over-stimulation.

Cannabis indica and Cannabis sativa

Cannabis indica when grown in the West alters slightly in its character-istics, and in this form is known as *Cannabis sativa*, which is also available as a homoeopathic remedy and appears separately in the refer-ence books. This western variety seems to have the exalted mental symptoms to a lesser degree, and the physical disorders more intensely. From this experience, homoeopaths sometimes use *Cannabis sativa* for the physical conditions when they occur.

CANTHARIS, canth

Remedy source: insect—Spanish fly.

Main uses

Cantharis is mostly used in short-term situations, usually involving burning pains. It is occasionally given as a constitutional remedy, although it is indicated by a few very characteristic individual symptoms rather than a well-developed psychological profile.

Acute uses

Cystitis. In some self-help manuals cantharis is presented as *the* remedy for cystitis. In fact it will only be effective in those cases where there is a frequent urge to urinate, and only a little is passed each time, and the urine passes drop by drop and stings intensely as it passes along the urethra. In some cases there are traces of blood in the urine. And the mood of the patient is one of heated irritability; even if all the physical symptoms were present, a placid, weepy patient would be most unlikely to benefit from cantharis.

Burns. Cantharis will relieve the pain of burns during the first few days following the injury. The cases which respond best to cantharis are quite severe, where the area is deep, angry red or even bluish. This includes scalds and sunburn.

Skin eruptions and allergic reactions. Any such situation, characterised by the intense burning pains, and angry, dark red appearance, may be relieved by cantharis, particularly if some of the psychological features noted below are present. A peculiar and strong symptom is great thirst with any complaint, but aversion to drinks.

Constitutional uses

Sexual desire, very strong and almost insatiable, is very characteristic of cantharis individuals. They are prone to problems in the urinary and genital area, including episodes of acute cystitis, and burning eruptions and reactions which are made worse by touch. The symptoms and temper of the patient come on quickly and violently. They are very hot individuals, worse for heat and better for cool applications.

Other remedy types with strong sexuality include apis, hyoscyamus, lachesis and platina. Cantharis seems to lack the emotional and psychological complexities found in such types, and just has overwhelmingly powerful sexual desire. If this is a feature of the constitutional case, cantharis should be considered carefully, otherwise it is unlikely to be needed.

CARBO VEGETABALIS, carbo veg, carb-v

Remedy source: wood—charcoal.

Main uses

This is a widely used remedy, mostly for acute, short-term conditions. There is a sort of chronic carbo veg picture as well, which is often simply a development of the acute condition if that is maintained for a long time and allowed to take hold of the metabolism.

Characteristics
The fact that the remedy is made from charcoal provides an easy way to remember many of the most important symptoms. The patient is

lifeless through lack of oxygenation—the situation could range from mildly lifeless after a binge, to nearly dead from drowning or the effects of a severe and prolonged illness. Just like charcoal embers, the patient is inert and cold but wants air, even wanting to be fanned. It is one of the most important remedies for collapse. If a patient for whatever reason is very weak and lifeless, clammy, cold to the touch although apparently wanting air as above, perhaps going blue, carbo veg is very likely the best remedy. It may be the one to give until medical aid arrives.

It is also a wonderful remedy for stomach and abdomen problems where there is a lot of wind, which may be passing up or down, or be trapped. The abdomen is distended, there is constipation with little or no urge and lots of wind.

Chronic or constitutional symptoms

The chronic picture is again characterised by failure of oxygenation. This may lead to constant or repeated digestive problems like those noted above, with sluggishness throughout the system, much flatulence and constipation. Or lack of oxygen may cause problems in any part of the body. Ulcerations in the elderly are fundamentally a circulation problem, and often carbo veg for a period will improve matters considerably.

The patient's condition is one of weakness, heaviness and coldness, with the odd desire for lots of fresh air, even fanning. If he can pass wind this brings marked relief, at least temporarily. Other clear indications of the carbo veg state are that symptoms and discomfort are worse for heat, particularly hot, damp weather; and tight clothing also aggravates intensely.

In a true carbo veg constitutional situation the fear of extinction emerges in other ways. The individual becomes afraid of the dark, and even of ghosts. In the early stages the mental state is simply one of inertia, with the patient lacking the energy to do anything and in particular to make decisions.

CARCINOSIN, carc

Remedy source: see nosodes, p. 197.

Main uses

Carcinosin is usually used as a constitutional type, and sometimes for specific conditions resembling glandular fever or chronic fatigue.

The constitutional type

Carcinosin is a very interesting remedy. It has only recently become widely used, and is a good example of how homoeopathy evolves according to the needs of time. The really characteristic feature of this remedy is not so much a particular symptom or combination of symptoms but rather a peculiar lack of symptoms, both physically and psychologically. Carcinosin is often indicated in cases of conditions such as glandular fever, M.E. and post-viral syndrome, and thus it is quickly becoming one of the most important remedies in modern practice.

Carcinosin types appear refined, sympathetic, fastidious, and have a strong sense of duty. A carcinosin individual will look after other people with idealistic intensity, whether the relationship is personal or professional. Concern for the other is selfless to the point that these types forget their own needs. They are fastidious about the care and organisation that they feel obliged to put into their duties. At the same time they are mild, yielding people, who hardly ever get really angry, or sad, or happy. They do not dream. Often their affections are directed towards animals, particularly beautiful ones. They love to travel and to dance.

What seems to connect and explain these features is an unfortunate disconnection from real inner needs. There is commonly a history of psychological domination during childhood, although this may have taken very subtle forms, and individuals go on to inhabit unfulfilling situations all their lives without complaint or even realising that things could be otherwise. They have been impelled to more than just a mature detachment from the lower forms of egotism, and are in danger of losing contact with the genuine needs that enrich individuals and cultures. They seem caring and committed, but in fact are beginning to live entirely in externals, in opinions and appearances. Psychologically they are becoming so divorced from themselves that life can neither challenge nor develop them, while physically they are vulnerable to the peculiarly modern type of disease without symptoms, such as the many forms of chronic fatigue. Examples of these depleted, selfless people, whom fate may reward with early death by cancer, are tragically familiar. If there could ever be a remedy for the condition of post-modernity, this is it.

However, the refinement of carcinosin individuals is real. They often have an unusual capacity for reflective self-examination, and for change.

Particular symptoms
A history of glandular fever or chronic fatigue in any form, and of sleeplessness in childhood. Lots of moles. Symptoms are markedly better or worse beside the sea. An extreme love of chocolate, may be present, or a fear of dogs and, especially, of spiders in otherwise sensible people. There is likely to be a family history of cancer.

Carcinosin may be given, successfully, in cases of glandular fever or chronic fatigue, with few or none of the personality traits noted above. See also the section on nosodes p. 197.

CARDUUS MARIANUS, carduus mar, card-m

Remedy source: plant—St Mary's thistle, milk thistle.

Main uses

Carduus is almost always used in conditions where most of the symptoms are centred in the liver, such as acute hepatitis.

Characteristics
Pain is around the region of the liver itself—the referred pain to the shoulder-blades typical of chelidonium is not present. Another very characteristic symptom is light or 'clay-coloured' stools. If such symptoms are present in acute liver disorders, carduus is likely to be indicated. Other symptoms that point towards it are that the pain is made worse when the patient lies on the left side, and on moving. The tongue is coated white down the centre and red at the edges.

CAULOPHYLLUM, caul

Remedy source: plant—blue cohosh, squaw root.

This is almost always used as a specific remedy in childbirth, taken for its power to dramatically reduce the length and discomfort of labour. It was derived from herbalism and folklore, and has been found to work very well in homoeopathic potencies.

It has one other specific use: as a remedy for arthritic pains in the fingers.

CAUSTICUM, caust

Remedy source: prepared from lime and potassium sulphate, according to the best laboratory techniques of Hahnemann's time.

Main uses

This remedy has some specific uses and is also a constitutional type.

Specific uses
Coughs, with a feeling of something in the throat but inability to bring it up. Causticum is one of the most-used remedies for acute coughs and throat infections with loss of voice.
Urinary tract problems. Cystitis. Occasional involuntary urination.
Burns. To relieve pain and promote healing after severe burns.

The constitutional type

Causticum individuals are intensely sympathetic people. They also have strong feelings of right and wrong, which can lead to political or social activism and even a revolutionary attitude. They are not necessarily easy people to get along with because their ideas of good and bad are strong and fixed and colour all that they say and do. While they are relatively well balanced this leads to practical, constructive action. When excessive or ossified it becomes divisive and hurtful to themselves and those around them. Their emotional sensitivity atrophies, leaving only vehement opinions. At an advanced stage they develop compulsive disorders, irrationally checking innumerable times that they have fulfilled little duties, such as locking the front door.

Physical conditions
There is a parallel loss of control and mobility on the physical level. The individual suffers from what the textbooks call gradual paralysis, starting with numbness, tremors and loss of control, and progressing to severe muscular and neurological disorders. Causticum is the leading remedy for Bell's palsy, especially on the right side. Arthritis and rheumatism develop, particularly in the smaller joints. The first symp-

toms may be a highly typical sensation that the muscles are becoming contracted.

Their other weak points are the urinary system, larynx and chest, with a tendency to flare-ups of the acute problems noted above. Characteristically they have many moles or warts, particularly on the face. They are chilly individuals but they do not like dry conditions, and are more comfortable in damp, moist weather.

In an interesting parallel to their intense sympathy but dislike of sentimentality and combative outlook, causticum types often actively dislike sweet foods. They do like pungent tastes, such as cheese and smoked things.

Causticum and phosphorus

See the note on the relationship between these two, in the section on phosphorus, p. 202.

CHAMOMILLA, cham

Remedy source: plant—chamomile.

Main uses

Specifically for pain, and for irritability. Teething is the most common use of this remedy, which belongs in the first aid box of every home with young children.

Characteristics

The most important symptom of patients requiring chamomilla is bad temper. The pains and discomfort do not make them weepy or frightened, but really cross. They cry and scream without restraint about the pain, and the only thing that calms them is to be carried around. Just rocking or rubbing or anything else is not enough, they have to be carried, and continuously. If this symptom is present, chamomilla is almost certainly the remedy; if not, it will do little good.

Other symptoms that confirm it include bright red cheeks, in particular one red cheek. There is diarrhoea, often with green stool. The state of mind is generally very capricious, the patient demanding something and then throwing it away, or not wanting to be spoken to.

Apart from teething, other conditions that might require chamomilla include fevers or upset stomachs with such symptoms; also colic, if colocynth does not help and the state of mind is present. It is indicated for earaches where there is much pain, no discharge, and the characteristic ill-humour.

Chamomilla is rarely considered a constitutional type, although adults looking after chamomilla children are likely to find it helpful when the same capricious temper builds up. It generally corresponds to anger, or ailments from anger, of the kind brought on by impossible people, rather than real tragedy. Too much coffee can induce or aggravate the chamomilla condition.

CHELIDONIUM MAJUS, chelidonium, chel

Remedy source: plant—greater celandine.

Main uses

Chelidonium mostly affects the liver, and is almost always given either in acute situations where the symptoms are centred on that organ, or sometimes to strengthen the liver specifically while other remedies are given in between or alongside it for more general conditions.

Symptoms
A common symptom of liver troubles is pain referred to a point between the shoulder-blades, and the most characteristic symptom of chelidonium is a nagging pain on the inside edge of the right shoulder-blade. Otherwise, there may be pain in the region of the liver itself, in the upper right quarter of the abdomen, perhaps extending to the back. Actual jaundice may be observable. There may be nausea, even headaches, where the characteristic symptoms indicate liver troubles as well. Sometimes symptoms are observed to get worse around 4 a.m. or 4 p.m.

Chelidonium and lycopodium
Liver troubles, right-sided symptoms generally, and symptoms worse at 4 p.m., are strikingly similar to the symptoms of lycopodium. The two remedies are closely related. The lycopodium type has a complex but well-confirmed personality profile, including a deep insecurity and superficial haughtiness, as well as the constitutional predisposition to digestive and metabolic problems. It has been observed that in conditions requiring chelidonium the metabolic imbalances have culminated

in frank disorder of the liver itself, and the state of mind is, if anything, simply domineering.

CHIMAPHILA UMBELLATA, chimaphila, chim

Remedy source: plant—pipsissewa

Main uses

Homoeopathically this remedy is used almost exclusively in cases of prostrate enlargement. Distinguishing between it and sabal serrulata is, in practice, largely a matter of trial and error.

CHINA OFFICINALIS, china, chin

Remedy source: plant—*Cinchona officinalis*, Peruvian bark, quinine.

Main uses

This remedy has some important acute applications, and there is also a quite well-understood constitutional type.

Specific conditions
China is very often used homoeopathically during or after acute diseases or injuries where there is great weakness, and especially if a lot of fluids have been lost, for example through bleeding or long bouts of diarrhoea, resulting in anaemia. As the source of the remedy would suggest, it is important in the treatment of severe feverish diseases, including malaria. (While translating a work on medicinal substances, Dr Hahnemann noted the similarity between the symptoms of malaria and quinine poisoning, and in a moment of insight homoeopathy was born.)

Gastric problems, with much bloating and flatulence, respond to it. A characteristic feature is that passing wind does not bring much relief. Conditions needing china are usually not so much the result of gross overindulgence as general sensitivity of the constitution. In such cases some of the mental symptoms associated with the constitutional type as sketched below are usually present.

China and some of its compounds are often used in cases of tinnitus, and also for headaches, relieved by hard pressure.

The constitutional type

These are very sensitive individuals. The beauty or ugliness of things affects them powerfully, making them vulnerable and thus apparently reserved with people they do not know well. They easily take offence. China people have a tendency to see themselves as unfortunate, and victims of the personal ill-will of others.

For the china mind, with its intense sensibilities, nothing just is as it is, and they read great significance into even little things—particularly into their own psychological processes. This brings refinement and insight if it remains reasonably well balanced, and tedious self-obsession if it is exaggerated. China types typically do not like to have animals around them, and often they fear dogs.

Physical symptoms
In an interesting parallel with their mental orderliness, their physical symptoms also show a marked tendency to recur at very regular intervals. Most typical is that symptoms flare up every second day. Mentally and physically china people are aggravated by superficial contact, and comforted by deep pressure. They are physically very sensitive as well, for example to pain and light and sound. They are very chilly people, and particularly aggravated by damp. Typical is a strong desire for tea.

CICUTA, cic

Remedy source: plant—cow-bane, water hemlock.

Main uses

This remedy is used almost exclusively as a specific treatment for convulsions, and sometimes for head injuries. A constitutional personality profile is not known. An odd symptom is a strong, almost compulsive, desire to go home.

CINA

Remedy source: plant—*Artemisia maritima*, wormseed.

Main uses

This remedy is usually given in fairly short-term situations, especially worms in children and animals. The mental symptoms are strong, and if a patient exhibited them intensely or long enough the condition could be considered a constitutional one.

Symptoms
Furious irritability is the main symptom of cina. The patient is at least as cross as the one needing chamomilla, and cina is a tormented, bloody-minded, hideously ugly mood. The individual cannot be consoled or reasoned with, and heeds no authority. He strikes out and breaks things, displays the utmost caprice.

This mood is often observed in cases of worm infestation, and cina is one of the most important remedies for that problem. Another typical symptom of both infestation and the cina state is picking the nose, continuously and energetically. The patient is also ravenously hungry, and prefers to lie on the abdomen.

Cina may be indicated in conditions apart from worms, such as infections or gastric troubles, or for the psychologically disturbed individual, particularly children, where the characteristic symptoms are present.

CINERARIA MARITIMA, cine

Remedy source: plant—Dusty Miller.

The juice of this plant has one specific use in homoeopathy, the treatment of cataracts. It is almost always the mother tincture that is used, diluted and applied directly to the eyes.

COCA

Remedy source: plant—cocaine.

Main uses

Homoeopathically this remedy has one main specific use—to relieve the symptoms of altitude sickness. Anecdotal evidence suggests that in this it is remarkably effective.

Perhaps surprisingly, this is not a commonly used or well-understood constitutional type. Some characteristics have been noted, one of which is a fear of falling. Some literature has noted great timidity of mind. Very typical is the sensation of creatures crawling on the skin. It has been used successfully for breathlessness in athletes and old people.

COCCULUS INDICA

Remedy source: plant—the dried fruits of *Anamirta cocculus*, kakamari.

Uses

Cocculus is quite widely used as an acute remedy, and occasionally as a constitutional one.

Acute conditions

Motion sickness. Cocculus is very often effective in treating or preventing sickness in cars, boats and planes.

Jet-lag. Cases of jet-lag with the general sense of disorientation and disruption of the body's time-sense; overtiredness. Effective both as treatment and preventative.

Nausea in pregnancy, particularly if the patient feels at all giddy or disorientated.

Vertigo, dizziness, for any reason. Perhaps after a shock, in unusual situations or during acute illness. If the vertigo is the main symptom, and there is no high fever present (in which case belladonna is likely to be needed) cocculus is likely to be the indicated remedy. It can provide wonderful relief to people exhausted and distracted by anxious nights awake caring for the sick.

Constitutional and psychological characteristics

In most cases requiring cocculus, vertigo is one of the main symptoms. If it is the strongest symptom, cocculus is one of the remedies to be considered most carefully. Often, the cocculus state comes on from a combination of debilitating causes, such as loss of sleep, long periods of caring for sick people, or protracted grief or anxiety.

With the exhaustion comes disorientation in many forms. Patients feel that time is passing too quickly, that by the time they have gathered their thoughts and their strength to do anything, it is too late, the moment has passed. This makes them notoriously averse to being disturbed or interrupted. And just little things, a light touch or slight noise, are enough to upset and irritate them. Although sensitive in this way, their manner is mild. Indeed, they are too mild, and are becoming incapable of expressing, seeking, or even realising what it is they really want.

In cases of grief a most characteristic symptom is a feeling of hollowness somewhere, such as in the chest or abdomen. Sometimes it is a sense of emptiness in the head.

Physical conditions
Apart from the vertigo, disorientation and exhaustion, they are prone to headaches, particularly in the occiput, and loss of muscular and nervous control. They are often further weakened by nausea from the sight or smell of food. And they are generally chilly.

COFFEA CRUDA, coffea, coff

Remedy source: plant—coffee beans.

Main uses

Coffea is used mostly as an acute remedy and occasionally, perhaps, as a constitutional one if the characteristic mental symptoms of the acute state are very marked and persistent.

Characteristics
The two strongest symptoms of coffea are sleeplessness from an overactive mind, and a generally overexcited condition, sometimes where the general disposition is happy or the cause is a happy one.

Coffea is often effective for occasional sleeplessness, particularly when the problem is one of general overstimulation, rather than fear, anxiety, or overwork, in which cases aconite, arsenicum and nux vomica respectively are likely to be needed.

It can relieve nervous tension and other conditions in children and adults brought on by a particular cause. The patient becomes generally oversensitive to any stimulation, and particularly to pain. The mind is constantly active. Any situation characterised by sleeplessness or excessive nervous sensitivity, and few other symptoms, may respond well to coffea. And most characteristic of all is what the reference books call 'ailments from joy'. It has been suggested that this remedy might have helped Beethoven with his nerves and hearing problems.

COLCHICUM, colch

Remedy source: plant—meadow saffron.

By far the commonest use of this remedy is as a specific treatment for gout. It relieves the pain of particular attacks very effectively and often uric acid levels as measured clinically are reduced by it.

It may also be needed for other rheumatic and digestive complaints related to uric acid metabolism, where the patient is very sensitive to cold and damp, to touch, and particularly to smells. The pains of the affected part are much worse on motion, and on waking. In digestive complaints there may be great distension of the abdomen, and the sensitivity to odours is overwhelming.

COLOCYNTHIS, colocynth, coloc

Remedy source: plant—bitter cucumber.

Main uses

Colocynth is mostly used as a specific remedy for acute pain. There are also some psychological conditions where it is indicated.

Pain

Colocynth is very widely prescribed for pains such as colic, period cramps, neuralgias and sciatica. It is perhaps the most-used remedy for colic in infants, in classic cases where the child curls up, screws up the face and fists, and cries out with the pain.

Adults describe the pains that have yielded to colocynth as intense, sudden cramps, or cutting, stabbing pains. They are the sort of pains that drive the person to press hard against the affected part, and sometimes warm applications are helpful. The patient wants to cry out with the pain. In this the remedy is very similar to mag phos, and frequently a task of the homoeopath is to choose between these two. If anything, colocynth is often worse on the left side of the body, while mag phos is the opposite.

Mental symptoms
The sense of having been stabbed extends to the mental sphere of what colocynth can cure. It is an important remedy for the effects of anger, and is probably sometimes missed at times when staphisagria is given. When anger or pent-up emotions lead to neuralgic or other pains, colocynth may be needed. It is anger of the indignant, outraged, mortified kind, the psychological equivalent of a stab with a hard, sharp weapon.

CONIUM MACULATUM, conium, con

Remedy source: plant—hemlock.

Conium is mostly used as a specific remedy in cases of induration or cancer where the physical symptoms are well established, particularly in the glands, such as breast, gonads and prostate. It also affects the nervous system causing a gradual paralysis, starting in the lower limbs.

The outlines of a constitutional picture have been observed. Most characteristic is a general hardening and gradual paralysis of the emotions, particularly in those areas where the feelings and sexuality are closely associated.

CRATAEGUS, crat

Remedy source: plant—hawthorn, the berries.

Crataegus is commonly used, and almost always where symptoms obviously stem directly from weakness of the heart and arteriosclerosis. The pulse is weak, small and rather irregular, and as a result of the heart's weakness the individual is breathless, prone to sudden loss of strength, to fluid retention, perhaps giddiness, and irritability. In some cases there may be stitching pains in the region of the heart or around the left shoulder blade. Also easy sweating.

Crataegus is said to have the power to dissolve calcified deposits in the arteries.

It is one of those remedies often used in mother tincture, and as such is one of the points at which homoeopathy overlaps with herbalism. Crataegus is often given alongside or in between other remedies, where the heart is under particular strain.

CUPRUM METALLICUM, cuprum, cupr

Remedy source: the metal element copper.

Main uses

Cuprum is quite widely used as an acute remedy, usually in situations where the main symptom is cramps or cramping pains. A constitutional type is recognised and occasionally used.

Acute conditions
Cramps. Leg cramps at night often respond well to this remedy. It also helps cramping pains that continue long after childbirth.
Coughs and acute asthma. The cough comes in violent spasms, making it hard to breathe, and in severe cases the patient becomes cold and blue. The attacks lead to vomiting, after which the patient feels better.
Digestive upsets and fevers. As well as the cramping pains the patient is very cold, to the point of blueness. Cuprum has been often used against cholera. One of the peculiar characteristics of cuprum is that symptoms are made worse by drinking water (this is a feature of cholera also). Patients report a strong metallic taste in the mouth.

The constitutional type

The chronic cuprum state is one that individuals grow into under certain influences, such as long periods of suppressing strong urges or feelings, particularly in celibacy. Things build up and finally come out in violent, painful spasms. Often nervous and muscular problems ranging from twitches to epilepsy are prominent symptoms of cuprum cases.

DIOSCOREA VILLOSA, dioscorea, dios

Remedy source: plant—wild yam.

Dioscorea is occasionally used in acute situations. The best-known symptom and by far the most common use is colicky pains which cause the patient (very often an infant) to arch the back, rather than the more usual response of curling up. This is the opposite of colocynth and mag phos, the most-used remedies for this sort of acute pain. Dioscorea may also relieve menstrual, neuralgic and other pains that are ameliorated by stretching out or arching the affected part.

Wild yam is used by herbalists in hormonal disorders. Homoeopathic ventures in this application have not proved fruitful so far. Disturbances caused by excessive ingestion of this substance have been resolved with homoeopathic remedies (particularly sepia).

DROSERA, dros

Remedy source: plant—*Drosera rotundifolia*, sundew.

Main uses

Drosera is a commonly-used remedy for coughs and respiratory conditions. There is also a constitutional type, although it is not very well understood or commonly prescribed.

Coughs and chest complaints
The founder of homoeopathy himself identified drosera as the leading remedy in the treatment of whooping cough. It is exactly indicated in the pattern of gasping and retching of that kind of cough. It is frequently prescribed by homoeopaths for coughs which are dry and loud and unproductive, come in violent paroxysms, and make the patient cough until he gags or actually vomits. In severe cases the coughing fits follow each other so quickly that the patient can hardly draw breath.

The cough is much worse when lying down, and most typically is caused by irritation in the larynx and comes on or gets worse after midnight. For all these reasons, drosera is very often in the first-aid box of families with children prone to severe coughs. Homoeopaths may prescribe it in cases of chest or even bone pains where there is a family history of tuberculosis.

The constitutional type

Features of the constitutional type so far noted include a barking, dictatorial manner, a sense of being persecuted, and the determination to achieve any given end. Appearing together in a single case, these characteristics have led some particularly skilled homoeopaths to prescribe drosera successfully for long-term conditions.

ECHINACEA ANGUSTIFOLIA, echinacea

Remedy source: plant—echinacea, rudbeckia, narrow-leaved (or purple) coneflower.

Main uses

Low fevers, repeated infections.

Symptoms
Echinacea is indicated in conditions that last a long time without coming to a head, such as low fevers or infections. Toxins remain in the blood and the patient is weak, tired, achy, chilly and nauseous. Warmth and bed rest alleviate the symptoms. This is the case in many disease conditions, but the feature that makes echinacea appropriate is that the symptoms do not change or develop. In this it has some similarity to ailanthus; with echinacea the focus is more in the blood and the glands are less affected. Echinacea is used to treat septic skin eruptions and other symptoms of blood disorders. The condition may come on after injuries.

Non-homoeopathic uses
Echinacea has gained a reputation for providing protection against infection as a 'booster of the immune system'. In the past such things were referred to as 'tonics'. Many individuals have expressed satisfaction with this application. If there are recurrent or persistent symptoms like those described above, echinacea may be used homoeopathically to treat them. If not, its use does not rest on the principles of homoeopathic medicine.

EQUISETUM, equis

Remedy source: plant—horsetail.

This remedy is used specifically for certain urinary complaints and usually for bed-wetting in cases where there is no apparent cause or any other symptoms.

EUPATORIUM PERFOLIATUM, eupat perf, eup-per

Remedy source: plant—boneset, thorough wort.

Main uses

Eupatorium is almost always used in acute conditions with fever where one of the most important symptoms is severe aching. No constitutional type has been suggested.

Symptoms
This is one of the best remedies for severe flu. The pains make the patient very restless, and are more intense than in cases requiring gelsemium or rhus tox; the patient says that the bones feel as if they were broken. It is the bones themselves that ache, rather than joints. Sometimes the pains are worst of all in the shinbones. The patient is very thirsty, very chilly and there is little sweat.

EUPHRASIA OFFICINALIS, euphrasia, euphr

Remedy source: plant—eyebright.

Main uses

Euphrasia is commonly used, almost always as a quick-acting remedy in conditions like colds, measles, other infectious diseases and allergies, when the eyes are particularly affected. No constitutional type has been described.

Main features
In conjunctivitis the discharge from the eyes may be yellow or greenish, and the eyes themselves are red and sore. In other conditions needing euphrasia the discharge from the eyes is clear, but it is profuse and burns the eyes and even the skin below them, while the discharge from the nose is bland. The eyes are sensitive to light. In some cases there may be a loose cough, which is worse during the day. The patient generally feels better in the fresh air, although wind in the eyes is aggravating.

Local application

Euphrasia is widely used to bathe the eyes if they are sore, itching and running for any reason. A good method is usually: euphrasia mother tincture, Regime J. This can be done at the same time as taking euphrasia, or other remedies internally.

FERRUM METALLICUM, ferrum met, ferr

Remedy source: the metal iron.

Main uses

Ferrum is surprisingly little used given the significance of iron in the wider world. In acute cases of anaemia, china and ferrum protox are more commonly given. When prescribed, ferrum met is usually as a constitutional remedy.

Characteristics

A well-rounded personality profile has not yet been identified, but there are a few well-known characteristics which draw the homoeopath's attention to this remedy.

There are usually signs of the sort of weakness associated with anaemia, or a tendency to obesity, and thus circulation problems such as palpitations, breathlessness and flushes of heat. Mucous membranes such as lips and eyes become pale. The face is red, making the patient look well and strong despite really being weak and vulnerable. Being still and exertion both seem to make things worse; gentle motion suits the patient best.

The remedy may be needed at times of change, such as puberty and the menopause. The weakness and changes leave patients unstable and overly sensitive, especially to noise and contradiction, and they desire solitude. They are usually chilly types.

FERRUM PHOSPHORICUM, ferrum phos, ferr-p

Remedy source: iron phosphate.

Main uses

Ferrum phos is very widely used as a quick-acting remedy in short-term conditions. Currently it is rarely used as a constitutional remedy.

Fevers, colds and other acute conditions
If a condition has just come on and few symptoms are showing so far, ferrum phos is likely to be the remedy (the other main possibilities are aconite and belladonna). Ferrum phos conditions come on gradually, and do not produce strong symptoms. The patient (often a child) is generally a little unwell: slight fever, slight sore throat, slight headache, rather subdued and miserable. The patient is tired, and better lying down, and usually wants to be kept warm.

Like phosphorus, discharges and mucus may contain streaks of bright red blood, but the anxiety and need for attention of phosphorus is not so marked. A useful remedy in earaches. The pain may be quite intense, but the redness of belladonna, weepiness of pulsatilla or inconsolability of chamomilla are absent.

FUCUS VESICULOSUS

Remedy source: kelp.

Main uses

This remedy overlaps with herbalism. It is usually used in low potencies or mother tincture for the effect of the iodine it contains in stimulating the thyroid gland.

GELSEMIUM, gels

Remedy source: plant—yellow jasmine.

Main uses

Gelsemium is very widely used in short-term conditions, particularly flu, and also in some mental troubles including anxiety. In cases where these are severe and persistent it could be said that the remedy is being used constitutionally.

Fevers and flu

Gelsemium is the most-used remedy for flu and flu-like conditions. The patient is tired, the whole body and even the eyelids feel heavy, there is aching in the limbs and back, shivers of cold and weakness pass throughout the body; the patient is slightly dizzy and disorientated, he feels dull and cannot concentrate. There is a headache and sore throat. The symptoms are not particularly bad, and gelsemium corresponds exactly to a moderate case of influenza in a generally healthy person. Dampness and humidity make things worse, fresh air helps. The patient is usually rather thirstless.

If any such symptoms come on just after receiving some bad news, that is a particularly strong indication that gelsemium is needed.

Mental symptoms

Gelsemium is used to treat the sort of mental conditions that come on before a big event, such as nerves and anxiety in advance. Other remedies have this, but in gelsemium cases the patient feels cowardly; he wants to hide away and let it all pass off without him. As in the flu, he feels weak, shaky, almost paralysed or incapacitated with the anxiety. Aconite is terrified, lycopodium is like a scared child behind the face of someone very grown-up, argent nit is assaulted by irrational fears; gelsemium feels that all his will is gone, he feels sick and floppy and will take any opportunity to get out of the ordeal. A few doses of gelsemium restore the man to himself, and all passes off satisfactorily.

The constitutional type

Agoraphobia and other severe long-term phobias and mental conditions with this sort of anxiety have been radically relieved by gelsemium. That the state was induced by a shock or bad news is typical. It is the paralysis by jellification that most characterises gelsemium states.

GLONOINE, glon

Remedy source: the chemical nitroglycerine.

Main uses

Glonoine is mostly used as a specific remedy for conditions where the main symptom is sudden surges of throbbing heat, such as hot flushes during the menopause; bursting, pulsating headaches with a great feeling of heat, and sunstroke. It is sometimes used for long-term conditions which seem to have been brought on by sunstroke long ago. The symptoms are slower to come on than belladonna, but they are worse and last longer. Heat makes everything much worse.

GRAPHITIES, graph

Remedy source: plumbago, black lead from fine drawing-pencils.

Main uses

Graphities is usually used as a constitutional remedy. Sometimes it is routinely employed as a specific treatment for the characteristic skin conditions.

Symptoms
Most cases needing graphities involve the stomach and usually the skin. Most typical is eczema or other conditions where the skin has broken and there is a discharge like clear honey. If this symptom is present, graphities is very often given so long as there are no really clear counter-indications.

Psychological characteristics

If anything, the mind of graphities individuals also tends to inflexibility. Everything seems dauntingly complex and difficult. They have the sort of mind that takes everything said to them very literally, and only later do they realise that things were really much simpler than they seemed at the time. Hence making decisions is difficult and the individual may be aware of rather lacking self-confidence. Graphities people may be moved to tears by music, particularly somewhere special such as in church.

Physical symptoms
An odd and rather typical symptom is weakness of hearing, which is less pronounced where there is background noise. Another is a sensation like a cobweb on the face. Physically, the skin (and nails) tend to thicken, harden and fissure. Most affected are the folds and creases, such as joints and the anus. Eruptions around the ears are very typical.

The stomach problems feel much better after drinking warm milk. Often the symptoms are worse on the left side of the body.

Generally, the type is heavily built, but chilly and very averse to draughts.

HAMAMELIS VIRGINICA, hamamelis, ham

Remedy source: plant—witch hazel.

Main uses

Hamamelis is almost always used for specific problems affecting the veins.

Characteristics
Hamamelis affects the blood vessels and particularly the veins. It is one of the adjustable spanners in the toolbox of homoeopathy and can be helpful in a great range of conditions dependent on veins that are weak and prone to dilate or break. As a result, the capillaries may become unable to supply enough blood to the area. These problems include varicose veins, menstrual cramps, injuries, even sight problems where the blood supply to the eye is impaired.

The affected area is usually sore, as if bruised. Warmth feels better, pressure makes it worse.

Specific uses
Bleeding. From the nose, vagina, anus or any orifice, when the bleeding is from veins (dark blood and oozing rather than gushing).
Injuries. To parts rich in blood vessels. Where bleeding as above continues long after the event.
Varicose veins. Congestion of the veins. During pregnancy or after standing for long periods, with soreness. When no constitutional remedy is indicated.
The anus. Haemorrhoids that are sore and bleed. Also, to repair the anus after large hard stools.
The eye. Veins swollen or broken around the eye after injury. If blood vessels break in the eye, hamamelis accelerates the healing and dispersion of blood in the area.

Local application
Hamamelis is used locally for its healing properties to the veins, rather than the antiseptic qualities for which witch hazel is noted by herbalists and others. As a cream or tincture it can be applied usefully to varicosities and broken skin in parts rich in blood vessels.

HELLEBORUS NIGER, helleborus, hell

Remedy source: plant—black hellebore, Christmas rose.

Main uses

Helleborus is a fairly uncommon constitutional type.

Characteristics

Melancholy, with apathy, is the main symptom of the helleborus state. The individual is emersed in depression and gazes vacantly before him. He can find no strength, no will and no reason to rouse himself. He is not angry or frightened, just empty. He is losing the connection even with his own body. Unless he concentrates, the muscles do not obey the will. And concentrating is difficult as he has no motive to focus his mind.

Sometimes helleborus is needed after injuries to the head. Long after the event the individual is still mentally dull and can concentrate only with great effort. Then helleborus will help. And it can be indicated in all sorts of neurological states, from headaches to palsy. The individual is chilly, and symptoms tend to be worst between 4 and 8 p.m. But what draws the homoeopath's attention to helleborus is the overwhelming apathy born of hopelessness. Many of Samuel Beckett's characters exhibit the mental state typical of this remedy.

HEPAR SULPHURIS, hepar sulph, hep

Remedy source: prepared by Hahnemann from equal parts of powdered oyster shells and flowers of sulphur, raised to white heat.

Main uses

Hepar is very widely used as an acute remedy in painful, infected conditions, and occasionally as a constitutional type.

Characteristics

In cases of infection or inflammation with pus or infected mucus, where the pain is made much worse by pressure and cold things and better by warm things, and the patient is irritable, hepar sulph is very likely to be needed.

Discharges are generally smelly. Mucus from the nose, throat and lungs is thick and yellow. Hepar is very sensitive to cold. The affected part is much worse for cold and the patient as a whole is chilly—cold draughts are intolerable. And the irritation is intense. No remedy is listed in the literature as more irritable than hepar sulph.

Hepar is often indicated in the established stages of infection. When redness and throbbing pain first appear, belladonna is indicated. Towards the end of the episode, when pain has subsided and stubborn infected matter remains to be dispersed, silica is the remedy. In the middle, during the stage of pain and pus, is the time for hepar sulph.

Infections of the ear, throat, teeth and chest, and boils, cysts and abscesses to any skin or mucous membranes, will yield to hepar when great sensitivity to touch and cold are present. When the amelioration from heat and horrid temper are also present, the remedy may be prescribed with particular confidence. The opposite of any of those symptoms more or less rules out hepar. Then close consideration must be given to mercurius, myristica, lachesis or arsen alb.

The constitutional type

A well-rounded personality profile has not yet been identified, but if conditions like those above are recurrent or protracted, the remedy could be used constitutionally. Chilliness, extreme touchiness, excessively irritable temper and tendency to suppuration are all features of the long-term hepar sulph condition as well. The individual has a craving for sour and pungent food and drink. A peculiar feature of the hepar mind that has been noted is a great love, or fear, of fire.

HYDRASTIS CANADENSIS, hydrastis, hydr

Remedy source: plant—golden seal, orange-root.

Main uses

There are a number of situations in which hydrastis proves effective. It is hard to perceive the unifying principles, and no constitutional type has been observed.

Characteristics
Hydrastis is one of the multipurpose tools of homoeopathy. It is often given unpotentised as the mother tincture, for its apparent antiseptic and rejuvenating powers, as herbalists use golden seal, and is one of the places where the two systems of medicine overlap. If anything, the patient is generally weak and vulnerable, at least more so than is usual for him. Warmth and rest feel good.

Specific applications
Profuse, thick, mostly green or yellow catarrh or mucus from the lungs or mucous membranes.
Sinusitis, where the discharge is more copious, less tenacious than that of kali bich, and the amelioration from fresh air absent or less marked than cases needing pulsatilla.
It is surprisingly often effective for occasional constipation, where there are insufficient symptoms to prescribe any other remedies with confidence.
Leucorrhea and vaginitis, with the typical discharge, lowered resistance, and few symptoms.
Cancer, as a support or intercurrent remedy besides constitutional and other treatments.

HYOSCYAMUS NIGRUM, hyoscyamus, hyos

Remedy source: plant—henbane.

Main uses

Most of the important symptoms are mental ones and it is usually given as a constitutional remedy, although certain causes could bring about a short-term hyoscyamus state in some individuals.

Mental symptoms

The hyoscyamus state is a sort of mania. The individual is being tormented. There is an element of personalised outrage in this condition; the patient feels their particular vulnerabilities are being maliciously assaulted. The result is shamelessness, obscene speech and violent behaviour, exposing themselves and their torment. Or there may be long periods of staring into inner space, sudden outbursts and great suspiciousness about the intentions of others. They laugh a lot, but the laughter is silly or inappropriate. All degrees of jealousy, sexuality, and loquacity, particularly in combination, are the keynotes of hyoscyamus. A fear of dogs is typical. Disturbed or hyperactive children, and betrayed or unrequited lovers, most often need hyoscyamus.

Comparisons
Hyoscyamus is less destructive that stramonium, more jealous and the passive victim of torment rather than its active agent, as stramonium is. Hyoscyamus is more hurt, less closed and hard than anacardium, and far more loquacious.

Conditions
Where physical symptoms arise, they are of the nervous system—spasms, tremors and nervous tics, even convulsions. Those who are embarrassed or ashamed may suffer sleeplessness. A dry, spasmodic cough is also a feature. Mental anguish and behavioural problems are its most common application.

HYPERICUM PERFORATUM, hypericum, hyper

Remedy source: plant—St John's wort.

Main uses

Hypericum is widely used as a specific remedy for injuries to nerves.

Symptoms
It is the main remedy for blows or cuts to the fingers or toes, particularly when they are very painful, and for the effects of injuries of the head and spine, recently or long passed, including vertigo and asthma. It alleviates the ongoing trauma of nerves, as when they are trapped and

in sciatica, and soothes pain after dental root treatment. Hypericum has also been used to treat other nerve conditions, including tetanus.

The pains are described as shooting, and they travel along the line of the nerves. Cold tends to make the pains worse.

Local application
Hypericum is widely used topically as mother tincture or in creams for its soothing and antiseptic qualities. It is often mixed with calendula for this purpose.

Depression
St John's wort is much used by herbalists for depression. This psychological effect has not been noted in homoeopathic practice, except after injuries to the head. And even there, by far the leading homoeopathic remedy is natrum sulph.

IGNATIA, ign

Remedy source: plant—St Ignatius' bean.

Main uses

Ignatia is very widely used as a specific remedy for the immediate effects of grief. There is also a well-understood constitutional type.

Acute emotional distress
Ignatia is by far the most important remedy for the effects of recent grief. It is not the only remedy that could be needed by someone who has just experienced a grievous loss; aconite, arnica, staphisagria and opium are among the others, but in the great majority of cases the remedy that should be given first is ignatia. What is really characteristic of ignatia is the feeling that one's usual coping mechanisms are exactly what have been taken away, at the time when one needs them most. It will relieve the distressing sense of being unable to believe, understand, accept and adjust to what has happened. It lets the gates open and farewells begin. It can safely be given frequently and in quite high potencies. Grief includes bereavement and other emotional losses like severe disappointment and the end of relationships.

The constitutional type

The constitutional type has often experienced a severe grief in his life, most typically the loss of a parent as a child or youth, although he may truly believe that the event is completely behind him, or may even have forgotten about it. Other losses at critical moments, and severe disappointments about the things or people one most trusted, can also lead to the long-term ignatia condition. In these people the coping mechanism becomes supercharged and they become exceptionally capable of dealing with anything. They are 'quick to perceive, rapid in execution', as the old textbooks encapsulate it. They set out to make good things happen, particularly for unfortunate people, and succeed in practical ways.

They become determined to see the positive side of things, to an extent that desensitises them to some emotional dimensions, and sometimes their intellectual convictions can get in the way of their hearts really tuning in to the needs of those closest to them. As the mind-set develops, the individual suffers self-reproach and a sense that his responsibilities have not been fulfilled. This drives him to pursue his moral convictions with increased intensity, and at this point the personality may become seriously unbalanced.

Conditions
If these people have physical symptoms they are likely to be on the functional level, such as hormonal imbalances and metabolic problems such as anaemia. Other characteristic symptoms are a tendency to eat for comfort, a sensation of a lump in the throat, and aggravation from stimulants such as coffee and tobacco.

A typical feature of the ignatia condition is that moods and symptoms change quickly and erratically. Pains fly from place to place, symptoms in one part of the body disappear to be replaced by others before one has had time to accurately record the first. And so it is with the ignatia state of mind as well.

IODUM, iod

Remedy source: iodine.

Main uses

Iodum is an occasionally-used remedy, usually as a constitutional type, and sometimes for short-term flare-ups of the typical chronic symptoms.

Characteristics
Iodum is used homoeopathically to treat conditions like those produced by excessive iodine intake and thus overactivity of the thyroid gland. The patient is restlessly busy, hot, hungry and thin. With this combination of symptoms, iodum must be considered very carefully, and the absence of any of them rather rules it out. Throat and chest infections, and allergic reactions, are found with this kind of metabolism. In some cases glands become swollen, while the body emaciates. The patient is driven to constant activity, not always constructive. Heat and inactivity intensify symptoms.

IPECACUANHA, ipecac, ip

Remedy source: plant—root of ipecacuanha.

Main uses

Ipecac is a widely used remedy for acute conditions, where intense nausea is the most important symptom. In particular if the nausea is not relieved by vomiting, ipecac is very likely the remedy to be prescribed.

Conditions
Upset stomachs, nausea in pregnancy, with the nausea and no relief from vomiting. Also respiratory conditions with lots of loose, rattly mucus in the chest, causing coughs that end in gagging or retching but without expectoration. Acute asthma, with loose, rattling mucus in the chest.

Other symptoms that point to ipecac include: being hot and aggravated by heat, thirstlessness, and a clean, even shiny, tongue.

Ipecac has also been used in haemorrhages with nausea, of bright red blood, most famously after childbirth. With developments in emergency medicine, that application is increasingly rare.

IRIS VERISCOLA, iris

Remedy source: plant—blue flag.

Main uses

Iris is almost always used as a specific remedy for migraines, with the classic symptoms of visual disturbance before the migraine, and nausea during it. Also for sour, acrid vomiting, during headache. Pain is often on the right side of the head. Lying down makes it worse; moving around gently is better. The migraines tend to recur at regular intervals. The attacks may be induced by eating too much sugar.

KALI BICHROMICUM, kali bich, kali-b

Remedy source: bichromate of potassium.

Main uses

Kali bich is used widely as an acute remedy for catarrh and sinusitis, and fairly often as a constitutional one.

Characteristics
The catarrh and sinusitis are very typical of this remedy. The mucus is tough and stringy and difficult to be rid of. It is yellow or white. Cases of sinusitis are often really painful, and the pain is concentrated in particular spots to which the patient can point precisely. Fresh air gives little relief. The state of mind is somewhat irritable but not highly emotional. The presence of these symptoms is enough to prescribe kali bich for acute conditions with some confidence.

Psychological characteristics

The true kali bich personality type is a down-to-earth individual, focused on the practicalities of life. Such people generally believe in doing things by the book. They can be reasonable, friendly, helpful and supportive, but for them the fact that a rule is a rule means that it is a rule. This trait has been identified as common to all the kali remedies, and it is perhaps particularly clear in kali bich.

They can be so consistent about this that it is a positive characteristic. In their case sticking to the rules is not a matter of being awkward or stubborn, it is simply their understanding of how things are. If the rules are changed—according to the proper procedures for reviewing and revising them, of course—then they are willing to alter their position accordingly, making them in many ways easier in themselves than other rule-conscious types like kali carb or lycopodium, who might be irritated and anxious respectively about the disruption to their personal positions.

The constitutional picture very often includes a tendency to recurrent catarrhs. Kali bich types are also prone to headaches, stomach problems and sometimes skin troubles, particularly ulcerations. Pain in small spots is a feature of all these conditions. They are generally chilly people.

KALI BROMATUM, kali brom, kali-br

Remedy source: potassium bromide.

Main uses

In current practice kali brom falls somewhere between a constitutional type and a specific remedy for skin and nervous problems.

Characteristics

The remedy has a few well-known mental symptoms, but they do not really add up to a complete personality profile. Most famous of these is 'a feeling of being singled out for God's vengeance'. Kali brom types have some of the conservatism common to all the kali remedies, but in this case there seems to be something of a moral conflict within the individual. They tend to have a relatively high sex-drive, and symptoms get worse at times of hormonal changes. The remedy has often proved effective in cases of acne and other eruptions.

Stubborn, prominent cases of acne that last well into adult life always call a homoeopath's mind to this remedy. If there are no clear indications for other remedies with marked effects on the skin, like arsen alb, sulphur and silica, and if there are any signs of a somewhat alarmed, defensive state of mind, and strong sex-drive or an aggravation of symptoms with hormonal changes, or at least not the opposite of any of these symptoms, the homoeopath might give this remedy and be happily surprised at how much good it does.

Religiousness is a common feature of the kali brom mind. Also a sense of being at the mercy of fate, which can manifest itself in nervous symptoms ranging from slightly neurotic wringing of the hands, up to convulsions. The nerves drive these people to restless activity. Kali brom types are generally quite warm-blooded, unlike other kalis.

KALI CARBONICUM, kali carb, kali-c

Remedy source: mineral—potassium carbonate.

Main uses

Kali carb is widely used as a constitutional remedy, and sometimes specifically for conditions including fluid retention and problems after childbirth.

Characteristics

It is often physical symptoms that indicate that kali carb is needed. Very characteristic is an aggravation of symptoms between 2 and 4 a.m. They are very chilly individuals, prone to coughs and colds, and hypersensitive to draughts. Yet they tend to sweat very easily, with the slightest exertion. Also common are swellings around the eyes.

Kali carb people have a strong sense of responsibility. What is right and wrong is central to them, and they are personally disturbed by what is unfair or incorrect. If these traits of character become exaggerated or inflexible, they start to feel insecure about their personal situation. They want lots of people around, but tend not to treat them pleasantly. The kali carb state of mind has been described as that of one who feels dependent on others and is afraid that they might not care for him properly. Unfortunately for those around them, and particularly for themselves, they react by becoming awkward, demanding and dissatisfied, thus creating the situation that they were afraid of, and producing innumerable confirmations of their fears.

Particular and physical symptoms
Back troubles are one of the complaints they suffer most. Another is fluid retention, in any part of the body. Kali carb has also been used to treat piles and asthma, worse between 2 and 4 a.m., and arthritis, with the stiffness of mind noted above. It is an important remedy during the menopause.

Kali carb has been effective specifically for acute attacks of fluid retention, backache and piles, without constitutional indications and particularly during and after periods and pregnancy.

KALI MURIATICUM, kali mur, kali-m

Remedy source: chloride of potassium.

Main uses

By far the most common uses of this remedy are in sore throats and tonsillitis, where there is a thick coating on the tonsils or tongue and few other symptoms; and in glue ear, which may be causing deafness. Otherwise the remedy is surprisingly little known or used.

KALI PHOSPHORICUM, kali phos, kali-p

Remedy source: phosphate of potassium.

Main uses

Kali phos is widely used as a quick-acting remedy, mostly for nervous conditions and exhaustion.

Characteristics
The individual has been depleted by illness or usually by overexertion, particularly of the mind or emotional resources. As a result he is weak, constantly drowsy and yawning, exhausted by little tasks, upset by small worries, oversensitive to discomfort, pain and cold. Warmth and rest make him feel better. The state of mind is miserable, preoccupied with his own troubles.

If someone is simply exhausted and mentally tense after a period of hard mental work, kali phos is likely to be the most helpful remedy. (If the patient is really bad-tempered and irritable, nux vomica should be carefully considered.)

Physical symptoms
In developed cases where symptoms have reached the physical level the patient is often hungry, with hunger almost like a gnawing pain, which comes back soon after eating. Discharges, including urine, stools, mucus and the coating on the tongue, may be bright yellow.

The constitutional type

In cases of long-term illness including chronic fatigue, kali phos has been known to help deeply, and just quite recently the outlines have been deduced of a constitutional type. Those who respond well have been observed to share the conservatism of the kali remedies, and the communicativeness of the phosphorics. The exhaustion and characteristic discharges are often also present in such cases.

KALI SULPHURICUM, kali sulph, kali-s

Remedy source: potassium sulphate.

Main uses

Kali sulph is fairly often used, usually as a quick-acting remedy for loose coughs.

Characteristics
The most typical symptom of kali sulph, and the condition for which it is usually given, is a cough with loose, rattly mucus. In some cases there is yellow expectoration, but often there is no actual mucus, particularly with children. The patient is hot and generally feels a lot better in the fresh air. In cases where pulsatilla fails to cure completely, kali sulph will often do much good. This has also applied to skin conditions where there is general warmth and thick, yellow, flakes. Good results have been reported on a constitutional level for individuals with characteristics combining the stoicism of the kalis and ebullience of the sulphuricums.

LAC CANINUM, lac can, lac-c

Remedy source: the milk of a bitch.

Main uses

This is a fairly uncommon remedy. It was quite widely used in cases of diphtheria, and is still given in some throat conditions. The most characteristic feature is that pains and symptoms of the throat alternate from one side to the other. There is also a slightly-known constitutional picture, of which the main feature is a very low estimation of one's own self-worth.

LACHESIS, lach

Remedy source: the poison of the bushmaster snake.

Main uses

Lachesis is one of the most important homoeopathic remedies, very often prescribed according to constitutional characteristics, and sometimes for specific conditions, particularly of the blood and throat.

The constitutional type

Homoeopaths consider lachesis wherever the patient is a warm-blooded person who talks a lot, rapidly changing the subject, with a forceful personality and strong opinions; and when jealousy is something to which the person is prone or has to combat, or in some cases actually indulges without apparent remorse. If the patient's symptoms are mostly or worse on the left side of the body, or start on the left and then move to the right, then lachesis may be prescribed with confidence. Predominantly right-sided symptoms almost preclude lachesis.

Other characteristic symptoms usually present, or at least not contradicted, in lachesis cases are an intolerance of any tight clothing around the neck, a tendency for symptoms to be worst on waking up, a great amelioration of symptoms with the onset of discharges such as the start of the menstrual flow, and blueness of eruptions and discharges. The mind, head, heart, blood, hormones, throat and skin are the parts most affected by lachesis.

Specific uses

Lachesis could be indicated without the constitutional characteristics, in inflammations or septic conditions or eruptions which are definitely blue, aggravated by heat or pressure, or worse on the left side of the body.

LEDUM PALUSTRE, ledum, led

Remedy source: plant—wild rosemary, marsh tea.

Main uses

Ledum is often used as a specific remedy for certain kinds of injury, and occasionally as a constitutional one.

Specific conditions

Wounds from sharp objects ('puncture wounds'). Ledum will help reduce pain, promote recovery and protect against infection.

Bites and stings. Ledum is often the first and most important remedy in these situations.

Bruising. Old bruises where the marks last a long time or even turn odd colours, and where arnica is no longer helping, have been known to yield to ledum. Often the most effective remedy for black eyes.

Joint troubles. There are rare cases of arthritis which begin in the feet and travel up the body, and where pains are made worse by heat and relieved by cold applications. If so, ledum is probably the remedy. Related to this is a weakness of the ligaments leading to a chronic tendency to sprain the ankles.

Characteristics

In situations requiring ledum the affected part is often bluish, feels cold, and yet is relieved by cold. This may be so in cases of bruising and conditions of the joints. In bites, stings and other wounds, what is most characteristic of this remedy is that the problem stems from deep, puncturing, wounds. This is enough to make ledum the indicated remedy in many cases.

Constitutional symptoms

Patients requiring long-term treatment with ledum have been observed to be cold individuals on the psychological level as well as physically. Emotional warmth disturbs them, and they retreat to solitude and ill-will. In some cases this condition arises in alcoholics. On the whole these observations have been drawn from cases with clear physical symptoms indicating ledum. It would be difficult to prescribe this remedy in long-term conditions without the coldness and relief from cold things.

LILIUM TIGRINUM, lilium tig

Remedy source: plant—tiger lily.

Main uses

This is a fairly unusual constitutional type.

Characteristics

The lilium tig personality is driven to constant activity. Being busy does make things better, doing little or nothing is almost intolerable. These are among the most hurried of types and begin many things, but finish few of them.

There is often a religious or moralistic element in the mind, of the kind that leads to self-reproach and agitation. Compounding this is a strong sex-drive, but mental and other symptoms tend to be worse rather than calmed after coition. The tension leads to intense irritability and anger, although at times the controlled side of the personality is uppermost. When angry the person is easily offended, and any comments or suggestions are taken as personal criticism.

Physical symptoms
Most of the complaints are of the female organs, nerves, hormones and sometimes the heart. Lilium tig people are almost always hot individuals, who cannot tolerate heat and closed places. Palpitations with hot flushing, and burning pains of the hands and feet, are typical. Symptoms are often on the left side of the body.

Comparisons
Like sepia, they are prone to dragging pains of the pelvic organs, but they are much hotter than sepia. They have many symptoms in common with lachesis. If anything they are less obviously jealous, more hurried and more prone to conflict with themselves, than lachesis.

LYCOPODIUM, lyc

Remedy source: seeds of the club moss.

Main uses

Lycopodium is one of the most important remedies. It is usually given as a constitutional remedy, and occasionally in short-term conditions, mostly of the digestive and urinary systems.

Constitutional characteristics

Particular features of the way a person's system works are what usually show when lycopodium is needed. The pains and symptoms are worse on the right side of the body and get worse in the late afternoon, between about 4 and 8 p.m., or the patient gets very tired at this time. The digestion is usually affected, with a lot of gas and bloating. The person has a sweet tooth.

Mental symptoms

Psychologically lycopodium individuals feel lack of confidence. They tend to react by projecting a bold exterior, which can unfortunately come over as domineering or haughty. In fact, they take it for granted that everyone is trying to stand up to the human frailties within, and that we all understand this. They are anxious about keeping up their performance, and suffer much with nerves before events.

Lycopodium types are cautious people. They take things seriously, and tend to frown, even as children. They may display a deep fear of personal commitments, in a way that seems out of keeping with their external respectability but which stems from the same source. In more advanced cases this can lead to really odd emotional or sexual behaviour.

The remedy is most often prescribed for men, but it will also help women and children in whom the intellect dominates, or who want to put everything into words and cannot simply feel their feelings. They gravitate towards jobs like teaching and administration, and often do well within big institutions so long as they remain fairly well balanced. If their traits of character become exaggerated they become increasingly exploitative of the vulnerable, servile to their superiors and ineffective in their work.

It is the right-sidedness, aggravation in the late afternoon, flatulence, frowning and love of sweets that usually suggest to a homoeopath that lycopodium is needed, and if these symptoms are missing it is unlikely to help. When the psychological traits are also present the remedy is prescribed with particular confidence, and often the result includes a happy lightening of the patient's mind as well as improvement in the specific condition for which he or she sought help.

MAGNESIUM MURIATICUM, mag mur, mag-m

Remedy source: chloride of magnesium.

In current practice this is a fairly unusual constitutional type. It shares the sensitivity and reserve of natrum mur, but with mag mur the unresolved emotions are quite specific: these individuals are very much concerned about violence and confrontation. Sometimes they will go to any lengths to avoid them, and they appear to be the most diplomatic, peaceful people. Alternatively, some are in constant conflict with the forces of disorder, in the world and their own minds. Or they vacillate between these poles. It has been noted that mag mur is often required by the children of fighting parents.

Physically, their weak point is the digestion. Milk may aggravate, and stomach pain comes two or three hours after eating. But it is a life dominated by the issues noted above the draws a homoeopath's attention to the need for this remedy.

MAGNESIUM PHOSPHORICUM, mag phos, mag-p

Remedy source: magnesium phosphate.

Main uses

Mag phos is very widely used as a specific remedy for pain and cramps.

Characteristics
Menstrual cramps, colic, sciatica, neuralgia and other nerve pains are all frequently treated by mag phos. They are sharp, shooting, cramping pains, made worse by cold and better for bending up and pressure, and much better for warmth. These are quite common symptoms and often the homoeopath's task is to differentiate between mag phos and similar remedies such a colocynth. If anything, mag phos tends to affect the right side of the body more. And the effects of heat are most marked in mag phos. Mentally the person is focused on the pains and talks of little else, but is less angry than colocynth.

Mag phos is also a remedy for painful spasms and cramps, such as writer's cramp and similar conditions, and sudden cramping in the limbs after much exertion. They are usually worse for cold and better for heat.

MEDORRHINUM, med

Remedy source: see nosodes, p. 197.

Main uses

Medorrhinum is widely used by professional homoeopaths, mostly as a constitutional remedy. In fact, medorrhinum is often more like an ingredient or layer, which presents at a certain stage in the treatment of a case (it could easily be what is uppermost at the beginning of treatment), so the characteristics are often 'themes' and 'energies' that colour a case, rather than the fundamental personality type. This is perhaps true of other nosodes as well, but it is particularly so of medorrhinum. Doing things to excess is very typical of medorrhinum types.

Characteristics

The true medorrhinum state is one of dissatisfaction, craving for stimulation, and disturbance of the nervous system. The individual feels that time is passing too slowly. The mind is too agitated to consider making inner adjustments. These people look at the world as a spectrum of consumables that do not deliver their promises, and they become rather cynical, and finally contemptuous. They may be sensitive and even refined, but are capable of surprising hardness, even cruelty, because of this feeling that things do not matter. A very typical feature of the medorrhinum mind is a feeling that everything is strange and unreal. But often they have lived with this sense for so long that they are no longer aware that it could be otherwise, and do not mention it at all.

They are troubled by fears, in particular a sense that something bad is about to happen. This anticipatory anxiety usually has no definite object. They are hurried in their work and movements, and particularly on their way to the next distraction. Their anxieties and urges make them averse to responsibilities, and avoiding them is one thing they do with a resourcefulness bordering on genius.

Physical features

Typical complaints of medorrhinum types include: chronic mucous discharges; pains, such as sciatica and in the soles of the feet; chronic rheumatism; skin problems; disorders of the reproductive and urinary systems in both sexes, and recurrent eye infections. Sometimes a personal or family history of pelvic infections is apparent. For some reason symptoms are much better beside the sea. Symptoms get worse during the day, but everything seems better at night. Lying on the abdomen feels much better, and medorrhinum children often sleep with their knees pulled up under them.

Children and other stages

Patients, including children, sometimes need medorrhinum between other remedies. Sometimes it is for chronic catarrh or pains which yield to nothing else. Then it is just a certain excessiveness, in the physical or mental symptoms, or even just a couple of keynotes like chronic mucus, hot feet, or the sleeping position, that indicate the need for a dose of this remedy, after which treatment proceeds again.

MERCURIUS CORROSIVUS, merc cor, merc-c

Remedy source: mercuric chloride.

Main uses

Merc-c is occasionally used (more frequently where dysentery is prevalent), usually as an acute remedy where bleeding from the rectum is a main symptom.

Characteristics

This remedy shares many of the characteristics of the other mercurius compounds, such as the vulnerability to infections. Merc-c has a particular effect on the abdominal organs, is slightly less sensitive to environmental factors and very prone to haemorrhages. It is often of great help in conditions with much bleeding from the anus, either alone or in between doses of other remedies.

MERCURIUS DULCIS, merc dulc, merc-d

Remedy source: mercurous chloride, calomel.

Main uses

Merc dulc is almost always used as a specific remedy for ear troubles. The ear is blocked, perhaps enough to cause loss of hearing, with wax or catarrh. There may be pain or discharge. Unless another remedy is very well indicated, merc dulc is often the most reliable remedy for quickly relieving glue ear and other blockages of the Eustachian canal.

The remedy has been used in conditions of the bowels, skin and mucous membranes, in line with other mercurial remedies. No constitutional picture has been described.

MERCURIUS SOLUBILIS, mercurius, merc sol, merc

Remedy source: a preparation of mercury devised by Hahnemann.

Main uses

Mercurius is widely used in short-term conditions, and also quite frequently as a constitutional remedy.

Characteristics

Inflammation and particularly ulcerations, dirty discharges, increased salivation, a metallic taste in the mouth and smelliness of the affected parts and discharges are very characteristic symptoms of mercurius. So too is great sensitivity: heat and cold, rest and motion, quiet and distraction—everything seems to agitate these patients and nothing makes them feel better. Their temperature is constantly changing and is never comfortable, and they sweat profusely.

Infected tonsillitis and mouth ulcers are perhaps the most common uses of mercurius. Also skin complaints, ulcers and abscesses, with thin, infected discharges. Ear infections, genital infections, and all sorts of fevers and childhood diseases often require it. The halitosis, salivation and sensitivity are what most often point to this remedy.

The constitutional type

It would be fair to describe mercurius types as mercurial. They find it hard to be satisfied with anything, and they feel that they have to be constantly on the defensive. They are perhaps the most suspicious of individuals; they cannot help assuming that everyone has hidden motives. Mercurius people often have strongly-held beliefs, and nothing can shake their fixed ideas. These may be of a radically political nature; in fact these views are the implications of their constant dissatisfaction and suspiciousness.

They feel driven by sudden, intense impulses. Being frustrated arouses the most horrible feelings in them, and they really feel like they could kill the person who has treated them like that. Often they are compulsive travellers. Concentrating is difficult for them and they become forgetful.

Physically they are prone to chronic or recurrent cases of the sort of conditions noted above.

Related remedies
Merc sol is a preparation devised by Hahnemann as a substitute for the corrosive mercurial salts used in his time. He used it for his own homoeopathic provings of mercury. He noted that the untreated metal element might be more easily available and that it could safely be used in homoeopathic potencies. In this form the remedy is known as *mercurius vivus* (*merc viv*). In practice, the symptoms of merc sol and merc viv are so similar that the two may be treated as interchangeable.

Where symptoms suggest mercurius and the main complaint is throat infection which is markedly worse on one side or the other, two compounds of mercurius are to be preferred: *merc iod flav* (if right-sided) and *merc iod rub* (if left-sided).

Mercurius and silica
See the note in the section on silica, p. 214.

MYRISTICA, myris

Remedy source: plant—*Myristica sebifera*, ucuuba.

This remedy has one specific use which is in the treatment of infectious conditions with lots of pus and pain, in particular abscesses. Sometimes remedies like hepar sulph, silica and pyrogen are not indicated or do not work well, and myristica will achieve wonderful results. Most widely used in tooth abscesses.

NATRUM MURIATICUM, nat mur, nat-m

Remedy source: sodium chloride, common salt.

Main uses

A very common constitutional type. Sometimes specifically for colds and herpetic eruptions.

The constitutional type

Natrum mur individuals have been emotionally hurt either by a particular event or over a long period, and have reacted by convincing themselves that feelings are not important. It is the leading remedy for the long-term effects of grief or emotional deprivation in any form. Typically, these people cannot or will not weep, and they hate fuss. Inevitably, their feelings cannot be denied for ever and they are vulnerable to episodes that expose their lack of real emotional resources, such as falling hopelessly in love with someone completely unavailable. Even when relatively well balanced they tend to dwell on sad or unfair events, perhaps in the distant past. They are sad and easily irritated by little things. Their interest in other people's problems is genuine, if not entirely selfless, and they gravitate to situations that involve responsibility and caring.

They react in a particular way to offers of consolation. They are invested in their sadness, so the suggestion that something as trivial as a few kind words could make a difference is intensely irritating to them, hence an aversion to consolation that is widely noted in the reference books. However, expressions of real communion and commiseration are deeply comforting to natrum mur individuals. Perhaps the single most common source of the natrum mur condition is to have had natrum mur parents.

Natrum mur types usually have a strong desire for salt. The skin is often dry and rough, and the hair tends to greasiness. Their symptoms get worse in the sun.

Typical ailments

By far the most common ailments of natrum mur types are headaches or migraine. They are so prone to headaches, and natrum mur is such a common type (perhaps particularly in Britain where emotional reserve is traditional) that the remedy is sometimes considered a specific cure for headaches.

Cold sores and herpetic eruptions are also common. And they are prone to all sorts of disorders of assimilation and fluid balance, which might have reached the stage of diabetes or hypoglycaemia. Dryness, of eyes, skin or mucous membranes, is a feature, as are hormonal, sexual, circulatory or skin problems.

Specific conditions
Colds, when the main symptoms include a thick white or clear nasal discharge. Cold sores, which come on in the sun. In these conditions the remedy may help where there is just a rather depressed mood, without the other constitutional characteristics.

NATRUM PHOSPHORICUM, nat phos, nat-p

Remedy source: sodium phosphate.

Main uses

Natrum phos is quite commonly used as a quick-acting remedy, and occasionally as a constitutional type.

Characteristics
Acidity and sourness are the best-known symptoms of this remedy, presenting as burning pains, acid rising from the stomach and sour burping. The metabolism is such that patients strongly desire fried, fatty foods. The tongue has a creamy-yellow coating. An odd symptom is a tendency to, or complaints following from, frequent seminal emissions at night, which are debilitating. The remedy is often effective in cases of worms, where there are colicky pains and perhaps the coated tongue.

Constitutional type

Good results have been reported for long-term conditions in individuals with the melancholy and sensitivity common to the natrum remedies together with phosphoric traits, as well as tendencies to the complaints noted above. A marked refinement has been observed in these types.

NATRUM SULPHURICUM, nat sulph, nat-s

Remedy source: sodium sulphate, Glauber's salt.

Main uses

Natrum sulph is a remedy for specific problems, and is also a fairly unusual but familiar constitutional type.

Specific uses
Asthma, where one of the few clear symptoms is that it comes on or gets worse in damp weather, often responds remarkably well to natrum sulph.

Natrum sulph has a wonderful power over the effects of injuries to the head. After falls, blows or even fractures, when arnica and hypericum have been given but can do no more, and still problems persist such as vertigo, even mood changes, and particularly headaches, then natrum sulph may bring great relief.

Psychological characteristics

The true natrum sulph constitutional picture almost always includes melancholy or depression. The person is profoundly sad and can see no light or joy in the world, only trials and duties. The individual thinks calmly and rationally about suicide. But a strong sense of duty and responsibility is another defining feature of the natrum sulph mind, and this compels the individual to carry on.

Natrum sulph types combine the grave sensitivity of the natrum remedies and the philosophic sulphur traits. They are the most rational of individuals with a remarkable capacity for detached reflection. Even if harmed or abused by others they reason that the other is subject to the drives common to human beings and that it would be wrong to be personally upset. So they carry on doing what they perceive to be their personal responsibility. The dark side of this trait is that with equal clarity they perceive nothing that is intrinsically good which would constitute the final purpose of it all, a reason for enduring all these trials and burdens.

Among the other suicidal remedies, psorinum types are tormented by a feeling that they are dirty and useless and spoil things wherever they go; aurums feel that death is the only honourable and tolerable course of action still available. Natrum sulph are the least emotive or theatrical of individuals, they can see only logical necessities, but no final justification for anything.

Physical characteristics

Physically they are prone to liver troubles, and to conditions of the head which for some reason are focused around the occiput. Occasionally they have genital complaints. They are generally warm-blooded types. All symptoms are worse for damp and foggy conditions.

NITRIC ACID, nit-ac

Remedy source: nitric acid.

Main uses

This is a fairly unusual but well-understood constitutional remedy. It is also sometimes used specifically for conditions of the rectum and other mucous membranes.

Characteristics

True nitric acid individuals are suffering from quite severe mental disturbance. They are never able to be happy and at peace and are always in conflict with the world. They are bitterly angry. Something has filled the mind with bitterness, and what has happened can never be forgiven—to forgive it would be wrong. They want to curse all the time. When someone is dominated by feelings of hatred, constantly expressed outwards at some object, nitric acid is considered carefully by homoeopaths.

The individual finds it difficult not to be absorbed in his own feelings. The tormenting dissatisfaction is always present, and it is hard for him not to be afraid of what people will do, and of dangerous diseases.

Body type

Nitric acid usually suits those with darker skins and little flesh. They are very chilly types. They crave fatty foods. Plump, blond, warm-blooded nitric acid types would be exceptional.

Common problems

Very typical of nitric acid, and sometimes present with none of the mental traits noted above, are complaints at the places where skin meets mucous membranes. Fissures and ulcers are most common. They are very painful, with sharp, stitching pains. Typical are fissures and other symptoms of the rectum including piles, with the horrid pain, and painful, bleeding warts. Glands too may be affected: swellings with sharp pains in glands, particularly close to their ducts, often require nitric acid. Gum disease is often a problem. Very strong-smelling urine is typical.

NOSODES

Most remedies are made from plants, minerals and sometimes animal sources. There is a special class of remedies that have been made from samples of disease material, such as germs and infected discharges. These are known as nosodes.

Constitutional nosodes

There are some nosodes, such as *carcinosin* (from a piece of cancerous tissue), *medorrhinum* (a gonorrhoeal discharge), *psorinum* (from a scabies vesicle), *tuberculinum* (from the lungs of tuberculosis patients) and *syphilinum* (the discharge from an eruption caused by syphilis, also known as *lueticum*), which have become part of the homoeopathic materia medica, with known characteristics and constitutional personality profiles like other important remedies. They are often, indeed usually, used in situations where the related disease is not present, although there may in some cases be a family history. See further comments in the sections on these nosodes.

General nosodes

The specialist homoeopathic pharmacies have nosodes prepared from many other diseases as well. Some of the most common ones have their own names (the measles nosode is called *morbillinum*; mumps is *parotidinum*; chickenpox is *varicella*). Others are known as *malaria nosode, glandular fever nosode* and so on, or simply by the name and potency, such as *malaria 30* or *glandular fever 200*.

These are used in two ways. First, to treat the condition itself, often in difficult or stubborn cases where nothing else seems to work. Although they may be something of a last resort, they are sometimes surprisingly effective. They are particularly widely used in veterinary homoeopathy. Second, they are given as a form of protection to prevent diseases occurring. This application is discussed further under Vaccinations (p. 113).

Bowel nosodes

There is a special set of nosodes known as the bowel nosodes. They are prepared from certain micro-organisms that inhabit the human gut and become problematic in high concentrations. Some homoeopaths believe that the bowel nosodes can eliminate toxins and improve the effectiveness of other remedies. One of them is known as *morgan co*, which is sometimes used alongside sulphur and related remedies in the treatment of skin and other conditions.

NUX VOMICA, nux vom, nux-v

Remedy source: plant—*Strychnos nux-vomica*, poison nut, noix vomiques.

Main uses

Nux vom is one of the most widely-used remedies of all, as a quick-acting remedy for many conditions and also as a common constitutional type.

Specific uses
Hangovers, upset stomachs, piles, constipation, fevers, colds, cystitis, menstrual cramps.

Characteristics
These patients are very irritable—the sort of irritability that feels one cannot bear fools and that the world is full of them—and really quick-tempered and nasty. They are generally oversensitive, with the nerves all on edge—hence the irritability and also excessive sensitivity to noise, light and disturbance. They are usually chilly. Sometimes the sensitivity means they heat up quickly as well, and then they are constantly pulling the covers on and off. Pains come in sharp spasms.

The constipation is the sort where there is constant urging to go, but nothing can be passed; and in stomach upsets they cannot vomit or belch completely. In fevers the back often aches, and the patient has to lean forward in order to turn over. The menstrual cramps are better for heat and worse for pressure. Cystitis is characterised by frequent urging, and is better for warmth. Nux vom is the main remedy for hang-over with acute oversensitivity and even delirium tremens. With all complaints are the irritability and chilliness.

Constitutional type

The irritability is their main fault. They have no patience with anything that they consider unnecessary or ineffective. They are fastidious types, with an eye for detail, and they are intolerant of other people's oversights. When reasonably well, the inner tension drives them to keep busy. Because of their focus on what works, and their fastidiousness, their activity is often constructive. They are never satisfied, however, and this undermines their judgement and long-term well-being.

Their irritability tends to make others rather nervous around them, and as nervousness makes people do things poorly, this reinforces the exasperation and irritability of the nux vomica type. If one stands one's ground with them they are quite reasonable, if not very polite. In fact, underneath it all is often an affectionate and generous spirit. One of the factors that can bring on the nux vomica state is wounded honour. When well, their honour is robust. The nux vomica constitutional type is a strained human being, but not a profoundly damaged one.

The inner tension drives them to stimulants: they are the type that could easily lapse into living on cigarettes and coffee. They are usually lean-built individuals, and dark-complexioned more often than not. They have a liking for fatty foods, which they tolerate surprisingly well. They feel much better for a nap (but awful if disturbed while sleeping). They have trouble getting to sleep, and then wake around 4 a.m.

OPIUM, op

Remedy source: plant—the opium poppy; the gum from the unripe capsules.

Main uses

Opium is used fairly often by homoeopaths, usually in acute situations, or where acute situations have made a great impact and become chronic.

Specific uses
Collapse. Opium is one of the most important remedies for fainting, collapse and loss of consciousness, nowadays usually given while waiting for emergency medical help to arrive. The defining features of the opium state are complete loss of all reactive powers. The patient is not particularly blue or cold or anything else, just totally

unconscious. A very typical symptom is 'stertorous' breathing—like snoring.

Constipation. Opium is indicated where there is complete inactivity of the rectum with no urging at all. The stool is just black, hard, balls.

Characteristics

The conditions that opium can cause and thus cure homoeopathically are notoriously difficult to understand. It is a remedy of contrasting extremes. Patients are either in a most overstimulated condition, or in absolute torpor and numbness. They alternate between intense activity with great clarity of mind, and the opposite.

An important application of opium is ailments after powerfully painful emotions, particularly severe fright, and shame. The patient is traumatised, and then follows the stunned, insensible state. In the energised phase there are delusions and vivid dreams. The positive and negative effects can be confounded—for example it may be the sense of fear that is anaesthetised, leaving a patient alternating between hopeless indifference and apparently rash fearlessness.

Physically there may be signs of neurological deterioration as well, such as physical numbness, loss of muscular control, convulsions and severe constipation. An individual in an opium state, acute or chronic, is usually hot and wanting coolness, perhaps with hot, profuse perspiration. Very typical of opium is that conditions that would usually be painful or distressing, seem not to affect the patient.

PETROLEUM, petr

Remedy source: unrefined oil from the earth.

Main uses

Petroleum is fairly widely used. It is usually given as a constitutional remedy, but almost always when the characteristic skin symptoms are present to some degree at least.

Characteristics

Most characteristic of petroleum is skin that is very dry and breaks open in painful cracks. These symptoms are markedly worse in the winter and better in summer.

A certain psychological dryness has also been observed in many individuals who respond well to petroleum. In the reference books they are described as timid and irresolute, and likely to lose their way in familiar places. In fact, while relatively healthy, they cherish realistic aspirations, and so long as those are fulfilled and others grant them the appropriate respect, they are quite satisfied. They are frequently successful in their endeavours in the long run, often more so than colleagues with compulsive ideas and fiery ambitions. Only when the personality becomes rather unbalanced do they become easily angered and confused.

Physically they are chilly people. They are prone to herpetic eruptions, and also headaches and vertigo which tend to affect the occiput, and disturbances of the digestion which are aggravated by fatty or flatulent foods. Head and stomach symptoms are particularly aggravated by motion, so much so that the remedy is often included in 'travel sickness pills', even though it will do nothing for the great majority of people who are not constitutional petroleums. (What they need is cocculus, which really is to spatio-temporal disorientation what arnica is to physical trauma.)

It is rare, and indeed difficult, to prescribe petroleum without cracks or at least dryness in the skin, worse in winter.

PHOSPHORIC ACID, phos-ac

Remedy source: orthophosphoric acid, *Acidum ossium.*

Main uses

Acid phos is quite widely used, where weakness is the main symptom. Phosphoric acid situations tend to be rather long-lasting.

Characteristics
Weakness or exhaustion with apathy and indifference are the defining features of the conditions requiring phosphoric acid. Sometimes they occur during a period of illness, in which case there may be profuse sweating or painless diarrhoea, along with the mental state. More often they come after a period of debilitating illness or overexertion.

Most characteristically, they follow an emotional trauma like grief or unhappy love. Perhaps the individual went through feelings of intense loss, but was then left with no will to struggle or even to care any more, and this is a condition in which phosphoric acid will help very much.

The mood is quiet; speaking is too much of an effort, and futile anyway. The eyes are sunken and surrounded by dark rings. Patients are generally chilly people, better for warmth. In the chronic condition, sleepiness during the day and sleeplessness at night are typical.

The remedy may be useful in children with growing pains, especially if they tend to overexert themselves and then go into the apathetic mood.

PHOSPHORUS, phos

Remedy source: the element phosphorus.

Main uses

Phosphorus is very widely used, both as a constitutional type and in acute situations, particularly coughs and chest infections.

The constitutional type

The phosphorus personality is perhaps the most extensively described, even celebrated, in the homoeopathic literature. Popularity is one of its main features. Healthy phosphorus types are the most affectionate people—to love and be loved is natural and simple to them. They understand how to attract affection: where the love-hungry pulsatilla child tends to cling and whimper until it gets attention, the classic phosphorus will perform, charm, do whatever it takes, to really arouse attentive good-will. One may be quite aware of the capacity for manipulation under all this, but cannot help forgiving it, even loving it.

Phosphorus people see things at face value, and this simplicity makes them perceptive about what people are really feeling. If someone is mentally suffering, they see the suffering and naturally identify and sympathise with it, rather than thinking about how the person may be at fault. They give warmth and sympathy, not advice. In this they are quite different from the other famously sympathetic type, causticum. In causticum it is the sense of right and wrong that is outraged, and they assume, often wrongly, that others feel the same way. Phosphorus simply feels for the person, whatever. See the note below on the relationship between these remedies.

Phosphorus individuals are prone to fears, especially of being alone and of the dark. Both of these aggravate all their symptoms. They tend not to worry much about material security or their relationships as they are fairly secure that the world will always be a generally sympathetic place, at least while they are relatively young. They do worry about the products of their own vivid imagination, and their health. But reassurance from an expert is usually enough to put their mind completely at rest. This openness to impressions is characteristic of the type. If someone presents with power and plausibility, the usually perceptive phosphorus mind may be magnetised, and left with no place within itself from which to make objective judgements. Natasha in Tolstoy's *War and Peace* is an exquisite portrait of the phosphorus mind at the mercy of its own lightness.

As they become older or more chronically ill, the picture changes. The love in them dries up and no longer arouses the interest of others. In this stage they seem reserved and preoccupied by trivia.

Physical characteristics
They are almost always thin-built people, chilly, and thirsty.

Conditions to which they are most prone
Chest complaints. The cough is usually dry, or with a little green expectoration, and talking or breathing in makes it worse.
Sore throats, with hoarseness and loss of voice.
Digestive troubles, such as vomiting and diarrhoea. They like cold food and drinks, and warm ones can make them worse.
They bleed easily and profusely.
The thirst, chilliness and need for reassurance and company are characteristic in all complaints.

Phosphorus and causticum

This relationship between phosphorus and causticum is interesting. They are two of the most important remedies for laryngitis with loss of voice, so they have to be distinguished carefully in practice. Particularly so, because the two remedies are 'incompatible'—to give them in close succession can stimulate very unpleasant reactions. And the two personalities also clash: causticums are among the very few people who do not get on with phosphorus types, and phosphorus cannot help reciprocating the feelings.

If one remedy has been given and it is wished to give the other, first administer one dose of nux vomica or sulphur, wait an hour, and then the other may be taken.

PHYTOLACCA DECANDRA, phytolacca, phyt

Remedy source: plant—poke root, American nightshade.

Main uses

Phytolacca is a quite widely-used remedy, mostly in acute conditions involving the glands.

Characteristics

The tonsils, salivary glands, lymph glands, and especially the breasts are affected.

Fevers and virus infections where the glands of the neck and chin are particularly swollen and sore often indicate this remedy. In all fevers and throat infections the right side tends to be most painful, and the discomfort is clearly worse for hot drinks. The throat is dark red, even bluish. In tonsillitis there may be white spots on the tonsils. Phytolacca might be needed in cases of mumps where the parotid glands are particularly swollen and hard; also in glandular fever, with the right-sidedness and particularly the aggravation of pain from hot things. (The person as a whole is chilly, and cold and damp can cause and aggravate the symptoms.) Often the patient requiring phytolacca has soreness all over the body, and it has been used in cases of rheumatism following glandular conditions.

Mastitis

The most common use of phytolacca in daily practice is mastitis. There are surprisingly few particular symptoms to confirm phytolacca in this condition. Sometimes belladonna, bryonia, or silica are clearly indicated, but if not, phytolacca can be given with considerable confidence. It is the main remedy for mastitis while breast-feeding, with or without cracking and soreness of the nipples. If there are actual signs of suppuration or formation of cysts, hepar sulph or silica are probably needed. Otherwise, swelling, heat, pain, and lumpiness of the breast often respond wonderfully to phytolacca.

PODOPHYLLUM, podo

Remedy source: plant—May apple, mandrake.

Podophyllum is occasionally used, almost always for diarrhoea. It is often very helpful in this condition, when the stool forcibly gushes out, and there are few other physical or mental symptoms. The stool is profuse and very offensive. There may be loud rumbling in the abdomen before the stool passes. Sometimes other symptoms including constipation alternate with the diarrhoea. It may help cases of painful teething, when the child bites the gums together, and has the diarrhoea.

PSORINUM, psor

Remedy source: see nosodes, p. 197.

Main uses

Psorinum is a fairly unusual constitutional type. It is occasionally used for specific conditions including skin problems and allergies. And, like other nosodes, it is sometimes needed to support the action of other remedies.

Characteristics

The true psorinum mind is in a wretched condition. Patients feel that they will never be able to provide for themselves properly, and will be forced to scrape along in a state of poverty. They are sure that the problem is in themselves, it is just the way they are, their fate, they are the sort that always gets things wrong. They feel vaguely unclean and even evil, not in a mad or sensual sort of way, but just cursed to be something that the world would be better off without. They display little anger and express few complaints, but they feel and somehow communicate that compassion would be completely wasted on them.

In an advanced stage the patient's mind turns to suicide. Unlike other suicidal remedy profiles, the psorinum type is unconstrained by a sense of being important to others, and is perhaps the most likely of the suicidal types to commit the act. Of course, the vast majority of cases never reach this point.

The skin and the mind are usually affected in cases needing psorinum.

The patient tends to emaciate, even if the appetite is quite strong, and to feel the cold. Skin complaints are itchy. A combination of itchiness, coldness, and weakness or melancholy that leaves the patient just wanting to stay in bed, is very characteristic of psorinum. The remedy could be needed in short-term conditions, or flare-ups of long-term ones with such symptoms. An odd symptom of psorinum is that the patient feels unusually well just before an illness. Apart from skin conditions, allergies and a general vulnerability to repeated infections are most typical of the psorinum state.

The psoric taint
Like other nosodes psorinum is sometimes needed in the course of treatment to augment the efficacy of other remedies. This happens where treatment seems to get stuck and there are few clear symptoms for any particular remedy. In cases where the patient has the sort of metabolism that is prone to coldness, emaciation and itchiness, even though other symptoms are not present, psorinum may do much good, and later other remedies can take up their work. In people with different sorts of metabolism, other nosodes will serve a similar function.

Such episodes are not uncommon in long-term homoeopathic treatment. They are related to a theory of susceptibility to disease, which Hahnemann called *miasms* (taints). He proposed that there is a fundamental human predisposition to chronic disease, which he called *psora*, and to which psorinum is related, although Hahnemann himself did not emphasise this connection. For those interested in this theory, see the introduction to Hahnemann's book *The Chronic Diseases*.

PULSATILLA NIGRICANS, pulsatilla, puls

Remedy source: plant—*Anemone pratensis*, wind-flower.

Main uses

Pulsatilla is a common constitutional type, and is very often used in acute conditions of the head, respiratory and digestive systems.

Characteristics

The most characteristic symptoms of pulsatilla are weepiness and the need for reassurance, bland mucous discharges, a need for fresh air, and thirstlessness. At least the first three of these are so often how people are when ill, especially children, that pulsatilla is perhaps the most-used remedy of them all in daily practice.

The Constitutional type

The plant itself is a delicate, pretty little flower, which grows in dry soil and moves easily with the wind. Pulsatilla's main defence mechanism is a vulnerability that elicits the sympathy and care of others, and on the whole it is very effective.

When mature and well pulsatilla types are aware that what they want is something strong to be connected with, and their natural sweetness and vulnerability often attract it. Although others might think of them as innocent and helpless, they are perceptive about what can and cannot be relied on, making them instinctively astute judges of character. They are described as mild and yielding, suggesting that they concede to the wishes and opinions of others, which they do. But it also means that, like the anemone in the wind, they can allow the power of forceful personalities to wash over them, without much affecting their own inner condition.

In line with the fluidity of their nature, pulsatilla conditions are almost always thirstless. One exception that should not deceive is that after long mouth-breathing because of the nasal congestion to which they are also prone, patients may seem to want lots of fluids. Their moods and symptoms change very quickly, like an April day. A good cry relieves many of their symptoms, as does reassurance, although it is probably the attention that helps rather than necessarily believing what is said, unlike phosphorus. Rich, fatty foods upset them. Stuffiness is the enemy of pulsatilla, and heat makes almost all their pains worse. On the whole they tend to be plump rather than skinny. Discharges are thick, bland, and often yellow or green.

If pulsatilla types become rigid or exaggerated, they lose their sensitivity and become just demanding and manipulative. They are as weepy and needy as ever, but responding to it becomes a chore. A sense of having been abandoned is most typical of the pulsatilla mind, and they hate to be alone. At worst, without support they are paralysed by irresolution.

Common conditions
Headaches, earaches, coughs, colds, upset stomach and bowels, menstrual symptoms, emotional distress, even varicosities and rheumatic

symptoms, with the mildness, tears, changeability, thirstlessness, thick discharges and aggravation from heat, will all yield time and again to the innocuous wind-flower in micro-dilutions. Such is the power of vulnerability. It was Hahnemann himself who first investigated pulsatilla's healing qualities: how he came to light on this particular flower is a mystery.

PYROGEN, pyrog

Remedy source: putrefied meat.

Main uses

Pyrogen is fairly often used, mostly as a quick-acting remedy in situations where the main symptoms are pus and infection.

Characteristics
The sort of conditions that need pyrogen are well-established infections. There is a lot of pus, with smelly discharges and a real danger of systemic blood-poisoning developing. In fact, if sepsis does take hold, pyrogen is one of the remedies to be most carefully considered.

Pyrogen conditions are less painful and sensitive to touch and cold than hepar sulph, less blue and sensitive to heat then lachesis, more putrid than silica, less unstable and sweaty than mercurius. With pyrogen conditions there are often red streaks, such as radiating across the breast or up a limb, away from the focus of infection. When the affected area is simply going septic, and blood and pus are mixed together, pyrogen is indicated.

Some flus and fevers need pyrogen. The pyrogen case is seriously ill, apparently full of poison. The patient feels a bruised soreness all over, making him very restless, as in conditions needing rhus tox and baptisia. However, the patient is more enfeebled than the one needing rhus tox, more septic and less delirious than baptisia.

RHUS TOXICODENDRON, rhus tox, rhus-t

Remedy source: plant—poison ivy.

Main uses

Rhus tox is used mostly as a quick-acting remedy for joint, muscle and skin problems, and for fevers. There is also a constitutional type.

Joint and muscle problems
Rhus tox is indicated where the pain is worse when the part is first moved, and gradually gets better with continued motion. It also worsens if the patient stays still or moves about for too long. This is so often the case with injuries and many common problems like arthritis and rheumatism, that rhus tox is one of the most used of all remedies. It will almost always help, to some extent at least, where the pain has this pattern. It is the first remedy for lower back pain, and is wonderful in back-strains from over-lifting, and in frozen shoulders.

Skin conditions
Skin eruptions like the effects of poison ivy indicate rhus tox. In practice this most often means herpetic eruptions. In chickenpox, rhus tox is usually given unless there are very strong indications for another remedy.

General features
The symptoms and the patient generally are much worse for cold and damp, particularly draughts. Equally, warmth gives relief. Rhus tox is indicated in flus and other acute illnesses where the typical joint pains are present, and the throat and glands may also be swollen and sore. All pains, including sciatica, are better for stretching out, and from firm pressure or rubbing. An odd and reliable symptom in fevers is that the end of the tongue goes bright red. The patient may have a strong desire for milk.

The constitutional type

The mind of rhus tox individuals is also rather restless and increasingly stiff. These people tend to be worriers, about things close to home, like the immediate members of their family. They are prone to superstitious fears, even if they know these are foolish, which are much worse at night, and particularly in bed when undistracted. If things get too much they can develop the sort of neurosis that forces them to repeat or check the same little thing many times. They are prone to the physical conditions noted above, and in most cases these are what draw the homoeopath's attention to the need for this remedy.

RUTA GRAVEOLENS, ruta grav, ruta

Remedy source: plant—rue, herb of grace.

Main uses

To relieve pain and repair damage to tendons, ligaments and muscles, where the problem is mostly due simply to strain or overuse of the affected part. Sprained ankles, torn ligaments, housemaid's knee and tennis elbow will all respond, as will eye strain after long, close work and pain or even prolapse of the womb or rectum after much straining.

Indications
Ruta should be given if the pain is fairly constant and the affected part feels too weak or lame to take pressure. Compare this with rhus tox and arnica.

SABADILLA, sabad

Remedy source: plant—cebadilla, cevadilla.

Sabadilla is quite widely used, mostly as a quick-acting remedy for colds and allergies, particularly hay fever where the main symptoms are attacks of violent sneezing, with profuse watery discharge and irritation of the nose and palate. These of course are very common symptoms of hay fever and sabadilla is often given routinely in that condition, particularly where there are no mental or other symptoms to indicate another remedy.

SABAL SERRULATA, sabal

Remedy source: plant—saw palmetto.

Main uses

This is the main specific remedy for enlargement of the prostate. It is one of the points at which homoeopathy overlaps with other systems of medicine. It is often given in low potencies, even the mother tincture.

SABINA, sabin

Remedy source: plant—*Juniperus sabina*, savine.

Sabina is occasionally used mainly as a quick-acting remedy where there is bleeding from the vagina, either for very heavy periods or for bleeding between periods, with bright red blood or mixed with clots. It is also given for a threatened abortion, especially at the third month. Typical is pain from the lower back radiating to the pubic area.

SARSAPARILLA, sars

Remedy source: plant—*Smilax ornata*, wild liquorice.

Main uses

Cystitis. In cases where the pain is worst at the end of urination, when the pain has not got up to the kidneys, there is no blood in the urine and there are few other symptoms, sarsaparilla is usually reliable. That is by far its most common use. A homoeopath might prescribe it for some skin or other urinary complaints, and sometimes for the effects of vaccinations.

SEPIA, sep

Remedy source: the ink of the cuttlefish.

Main uses

Sepia is very widely used, mostly as a constitutional remedy.

Characteristics

Someone in the true sepia state is drained, physically and emotionally. They feel they have given more than they had to give, or rather that it has been taken. They want to be left alone to themselves and for no one to make any more demands on them, for care or attention or affection and most of all for sex. If anyone does cross the line, sepia reacts with fierce irritability. In their emotional exhaustion they are acutely sensitive to exactly what people really want, and equally to their foibles and weaknesses. An irritated sepia is capable of the most penetratingly hurtful remarks.

They cry easily and often, particularly if drawn to talk about their ailments, although insensitive attempts at consolation infuriate them. One thing that does make the sepia individual feel better is if they force themselves, or are forced, to take vigorous exercise.

Another face

Often, and stereotypically, sepia is a domestic woman who has borne and raised a lot of children. As lifestyles change another face of sepia is becoming more familiar. Her inclination to be alone has kept her feelings withdrawn, she has avoided emotional involvements and turned her energies and attention to material concerns. Her perceptivity, directness, self-containment and need for intense activity make her very effective in worldly affairs. This type of sepia may be highly sexed, if emotionally cool. Only when unwell or unbalanced does she display the depleted state.

Physical features and complaints

When unwell, the sepia individual becomes physically static and congested. In the majority of cases requiring sepia, but not all, the hormonal system is involved. The circulation is disturbed causing headaches and varicosities. The whole pelvic area becomes irritated, and very typically there are bearing down pains, as if the parts would prolapse. Patients become constipated. The skin is prone to herpetic eruptions. For these complaints, with the irritability and need to be alone, or rather for personal space, when they occur or get worse during and after menstruation, pregnancy, termination or the menopause, sepia is a mainstay of daily practice.

Sepia types are usually thin-built, or pear-shaped, and do not stand the cold. They have an acute sense of smell.

SILICA (SILICEA), sil

Remedy source: pure flint, or white sand.

Main uses

Silica is very widely used, both in short-term conditions where infections are established, and as a constitutional type.

Specific uses

Homoeopathic silica has a remarkable power for expelling toxins from the body. Abscesses, when they are mature, not so painful, but where pus and toxins remain; and all kinds of cysts and infections, particularly where pus and waste products have calcified, are dispersed or expelled by silica. Often relatively high potencies are best for this work. Also in old infections, of the chest and elsewhere, where stubborn matter remains, and in sinusitis where there is much congestion but little discharge, silica will give great relief. It often follows after hepar sulph in active infections. Splinters and foreign bodies lodged in the flesh have been expelled by silica.

The constitutional type

True silica types are famously irresolute, and stubborn. They have terrible trouble making decisions: even having chosen a course of action, the mind discovers further drawbacks and they hesitate again. They remain in modest positions, where they do no harm and little good. They lack the warmth and strength of spirit that recognises nothing is perfect and acts creatively, ready to adjust with change and experience. From fear of failure, or rather from fear of being responsible for something of which they do not fully approve, they do nothing.

They are stubborn in their refusal to be compromised. Neither powerful personalities nor any amount of reasoning will convince them that they should abandon the stance they have taken, or come out of the shelter into which they have withdrawn. The silica mind chooses to concern itself with little things, and then does so with great determination. At some level these types are aware that this is a failing, and feel discontented and irritable with themselves.

Positively, they have an above-average capacity for seeing more than one side to a situation, and accommodating personalities very different from their own. And if circumstances present them with a specific objective that without doubt must be obtained (pass an exam, uphold a principle), they will pursue it with heroic tenacity. Silica types often have very active dream lives, and may be genuinely clairvoyant.

Children
Silica children often have rather large heads. They have trouble taking milk, even that of their mothers. Early on they begin to show the combination of mildness and lack of self-confidence, together with stubbornness about certain things, that typifies the adult.

Physical features and predispositions
Silica types are lightly built and often fair-skinned, and chilly. They sweat easily, particularly on the feet, which may become offensive. They tend to suffer with skin problems, repeated infections, fungal conditions, ear infections, weak chests, constipation and headaches,

particularly at the back of the head and into the neck. Silica bones tend to be fine and delicate. Problems with hair, teeth and especially the nails are very common.

Silica and mercurius

The exception to silica's generally tolerant nature is in relation to the mercurial mercurius, with which it is violently incompatible: the two personality types do not get on at all, and if given in succession the two remedies frequently cause nasty aggravations. They are both often indicated in suppurating conditions and you may have tried one and wish to give the other. If so, first give one dose of sulphur or hepar sulph, wait an hour, and then the other remedy may be given safely.

SOL

Remedy source: the rays of the sun.

The remedy is prepared by exposing a neutral substance, usually sugar or milk or alcohol, to the sun. Then this is potentised in the usual way. The remedy is exclusively used for conditions arising from, or excessive sensitivity to, the sun.

SPONGIA TOSTA, spongia, spong

Remedy source: common sea sponge, roasted.

Main uses

Spongia is used mostly as a quick-acting remedy for coughs. Because of the iodine content of the source of this remedy, it is sometimes used in thyroid problems and occasionally in conditions of other glands, including the testes. Usually some respiratory symptoms are present.

Main symptoms
By far the most important indication for spongia is a cough that is dry and loud. The spongia cough is often described as like the bark of a seal, or the sound of sawing a board. The problem may be diagnosed as croup or asthma, with that kind of cough. The cough is very dry, nothing comes up and there is little or no rattling in the chest.

Comparisons

Spongia conditions resemble those requiring drosera. Both have dry, violent coughs. Spongia is the louder, drosera is most likely to end in vomiting.

General characteristics

Cold conditions can bring on the problem, but warm food or drinks seem to make it worse. It has been observed that lying on the right side aggravates it. The cough often comes on after the patient has been sleeping for a while, frequently around midnight. But when the dryness and loudness of the cough are present, spongia can be given with confidence.

STAPHISAGRIA, staph

Remedy source: plant—*Delphinium staphisagria*, staveacre.

Main uses

Staphisagria is widely used, sometimes for acute problems but more often as a constitutional remedy. Usually the staphisagria condition is one that has arisen in response to circumstances, rather than an absolutely fundamental body-type that someone is born with.

Characteristics

Staphisagria individuals are angry—so angry that they throw things, get into screaming rows with people in the street, break things and swear. The one thing they don't do is direct all that energy at the cause of the anger. They cannot do so, because the culprit got away, or because they do not have the power, or because they cannot face confrontation, or because the person who hurt them does not care enough to be hurt in return. Anger is universal; it is the undercurrent of powerlessness in relation to the cause of their anger that is the really characteristic feature of staphisagria. The textbooks call it anger with or from indignation or mortification. Their person and integrity have been invaded.

Sometimes staphisagria people progress from impotent anger to submissiveness. At this stage they seem to be particularly mild and yielding, but ailments arise from the force of suppressed feelings. Frequently they gravitate to caring of personnel-centred professions. But the anger is unassimilated, and they are still prone to fits of rage that are as exaggerated as they are ultimately futile. And the excessive mildness is detected by others and tends to bring out a rather impatient, intrusive streak in them, to which the staphisagria can only respond with more indignation, or submission. Thus staphisagrias may get locked into mutually harmful relationships with impatient and insensitive partners. The individual who expects to be abused, and who understands no other expression of care, is the tragic end-state of this dynamic.

Typical conditions
Almost any condition that came on after being humiliated, mortified, attacked, betrayed, lied to, taken advantage of, abused, insulted, raped, or simply got-at for long periods, is very likely to need staphisagria where the indignation or mildness is present. There is often a sexual element, either in the initiating cause or in the way the individual expresses his or her frustration.

The physical conditions to which staphisagria individuals are most prone are skin eruptions, sties, headaches, cystitis, and irritable bowels. Most typical of all are problems with their teeth. Not only do they feel psychologically toothless, but their teeth become weak, discoloured or painful.

Short-term uses
The most common acute application is, as the old reference books gracefully put it, cystitis in newly married women. In this case, the mental state need not be present. On a physical level it can help repair and minimise the pain of deep cuts, particularly to the pelvic organs. It is a wonderful remedy after emergency Caesareans and hysterectomies. And the mother tincture is used locally for one of the most elemental invasions of all: head-lice.

As staphisagria is more of a state than a constitution, one cannot indicate a body-type or metabolism that is typical.

STRAMONIUM, stram

Remedy source: plant—thorn-apple.

Main uses

Stramonium is usually given as a constitutional remedy, but it could be used in acute episodes with symptoms similar to those of the constitutional state.

Characteristics

The stramonium mind is prone to intense fears. These are about violent dangers, and they provoke violent reactions. There is something quite demoniacal about this state: the fear is such that the normal restraints are removed and the individual is back in a condition of elemental fear. The symptoms may arise from frightening experiences, the sight of violent confrontations, the experience of danger, or even a diet of horror films and violent culture.

When subject to the fears, individuals are capable of violently destructive behaviour, sometimes to themselves, more typically to others. The child kicks and strikes, the adult fights, abuses, puts himself and others in real danger. Stramonium is an important remedy in the treatment of disturbed children, and in cases approaching mania.

In some cases requiring stramonium the violence is not yet apparent. So far, the patient has come to feel just danger, and the reaction has not occurred. Absolutely typical of stamonium minds is a feeling that they have been 'abandoned in a wilderness'. At this point the patient may exhibit a degree of vulnerability reminiscent of pulsatilla. With stramonium is a sense of terrible danger, and that there is nowhere safe to go.

Typical conditions
In general with stramonium states the full force of the disease exerts itself on the mind and nervous system; the behaviour may be severely disturbed, but there are few physical symptoms except functional disorders of the nervous system such as stammers or convulsions. Darkness and being alone make stramonium symptoms worse. Light relieves, although there may be a peculiar fear of shiny, glistening objects.

SULPHUR, sulph

Remedy source: the element from flowers of sulphur, brimstone.

Main uses

Sulphur is perhaps the most widely-used constitutional remedy of all, and is sometimes given in short-term situations as well.

Characteristics

It is hard to point out the central features of the sulphur constitution, because there seem to be many sulphur types. Some sulphur people are in a miserable state; unable to assimilate nourishment properly, prone to itchy conditions, and a victim of their own chaotic inner world. Others are marked by an almost luminous sense of integrity, and are among the most creative of individuals.

Perhaps if there is one characteristic common to all the varieties of sulphur it is a somewhat heightened self-awareness or self-consciousness. Others perceive them as self-conscious, self-centred or self-assured, according to the other's own spectacles. This I-ness is integral to the best, and worst, of the human condition. One well-known sulphur type is the itchy, lazy, pseudo-philosopher with an inflated opinion of his own intelligence and importance; another is a great-spirited genius; another is a warm-blooded, warm-hearted person with a passion for toffee and gadgets. Sulphur is given innumerable homoeopathic applications right across this spectrum of human limitations.

Common to most sulphur types is a tendency to think in a theoretical way. They are not devoid of emotions, but they theorise about them rather than just feeling them. They are rarely tidy and well-organised people, and are usually the opposite. Being theoretical they have ideas about what is correct and incorrect, and often express them. As a result they can appear haughty, critical and insensitive about others' feelings, although this is usually genuine insensitivity rather than malice; their theories about feelings, including their own, are often more of a distraction than an insight. An oddly common feature of the sulphur mind is a fear of heights. Related to their self-awareness is a tendency to be easily embarrassed, and to fear embarrassment. And they may be easily nauseated by bad smells and effluvia, including their own.

Typical conditions
They are most prone to conditions of the skin and the whole gastro-intestinal tract. Itchy eruptions, which are worse for heat and bathing, and itchy orifices, are very common. They suffer from headaches, particularly on the vertex, itchy piles and symptoms during the menopause. Certain parts of the body, like the ears or lips, are often bright red.

They tend to be warm-blooded people, although the skinny ones may be chilly. Their metabolism is such that certain parts at least get hot, especially the feet. They wake up with little appetite, but need sugary snacks mid-morning. An urgent need to pass a loose stool first thing in the morning is very typical.

Sulphur children
Sulphur children are fundamentally healthy, often charming, and a very common type. Curiosity and untidiness are frequently the main features of their minds. The babies (sulphur is the second most common baby-type, after calc carb) are drier and less sweaty and more prone to itchy eruptions and nappy-rash than infant calc carbs.

SYMPHYTUM, symph

Remedy source: plant—comfrey.

By far the most common use of symphytum is to promote the healing of bone fractures, which it does remarkably well. Even bad breaks, such as those near the major joints, and in the elderly and weak, can be healed more quickly and often without elaborate surgical intervention.

The literature records cures of bone tumours by this remedy.

One other use of sympthytum is in injuries to the eye, where the eye ball itself is traumatised, as by a direct blow from a blunt instrument.

SYPHILINUM, syph

Remedy source: see nosodes, p. 197.

Main uses

Syphilinum is the least used and least understood of the major nosodes. There are just a few well-known features, and a very broad, but equally vague 'theme'. Often it is one of the keynotes, a hint of the theme, and the fact that other remedies are not working well for no obvious reason, that draw the homoeopath's attention to the need for syphilinum.

Characteristics

True syphilinum patients are tormented by feelings of worthlessness. They feel dirty and develop an intense fear of dirt and infections, leading them to a compulsive, constant, washing of their hands or their clothes. This is the most famous of the syphilinum clues, but other forms of neurotic compulsion may also arise. Very typical is a personal or family history of self-destructiveness, such as suicide or alcoholism, and a general tendency always to expect the worst of themselves and the world. These individuals have been afflicted with great suffering, but they seem to want to prove that no one could be capable of feeling compassion for them.

Physical symptoms and the mental condition are much worse at night, literally from when the sun goes down until dawn. Also common are congenital defects, and destructive, corrosive disease processes, like ulceration.

The syphilinum trait
As noted above, sometimes other remedies are failing unaccountably, indicating to the homoeopath that one of the nosodes is needed for the 'unblocking' function that can be performed by the nosodes generally. Then it could be just a hint like the aggravation at night, or family history of self-destructiveness, that points towards syphilinum, which may do much good without the other features of the constitutional type being present.

SYZYGIUM JAMBOLANUM, syzygium, syzyg

Remedy source: plant—jumbul.

Main uses

This remedy has one main use which is in the control of diabetes mellitus. Many diabetics who monitor their own blood-sugar levels have found that syzygium substantially reduces blood-sugar, without apparent ill-effects. It may be used to good effect alongside constitutional remedies when they are being used to correct metabolic imbalances.

THUJA OCCIDENTALIS, thuja, thuj

Remedy source: plant—conifer, arbor vitae.

Main uses

Thuja is often used as a specific remedy, locally and internally, for warts and other viral eruptions. It is also a major constitutional type.

Characteristics

The nature of the thuja remedy profile is notoriously elusive and difficult to grasp. Perhaps that is the heart of it: the main characteristic of thuja people is that they are elusive and difficult to know. This is largely because they are consciously camouflaging themselves. What exactly they are hiding is elusive too; they suffer from a sense of guilt and shame, but usually without a clear object. What they seem to be most disturbed about is that others will see they are not being straightforward and sincere. This makes them uncomfortable in themselves. Physically, they are prone to the unpleasantly pungent perspiration and body-smell of the embarrassed. And their discomfort inevitably communicates itself to others, fulfilling the fear that their disguise will be perceived for what it is.

This might sound theoretical, but in actual practice it is often a certain elusiveness in the symptoms and character of the patient, defying attempts to make a whole of the parts, that alerts the homoeopath to the need for thuja, which may then be given to good effect.

Thuja people genuinely want to be genuine, but are afflicted by an unusually intense sense of not knowing who they are, or what they really think and feel. If this conflict can be resolved, a corresponding degree of refinement and insight is achieved.

Sometimes their lack of inner foundations leads to compensation, and another well-observed feature of the thuja mind is a tendency to fixed ideas. About certain, perhaps apparently unimportant things, they have weird ideas and theories, strongly held and immune to reason.

Typical conditions
Apart from the sweet-smelling perspiration, other typical marks of thuja include distorted nails, and a history of a tendency to warts. Yellow-green discharges are typical. Thuja types often drink very large quantities of tea. Physiologically they are prone to odd perceptions about their own bodies. This is on the border between what they feel and what they believe about their bodies. That parts of themselves feel delicate, transparent or alive are among the many reported variations on this theme.

Thuja individuals are most prone to conditions of the mind, skin and urinary and genital organs. Thuja is often given routinely for warts, where none of the other symptoms are present, and has some effect in a surprising number of cases (although probably less than 50 per cent).

Thuja and vaccination

For reasons no one really understands thuja is one of several remedies that have been observed to help resolve harmful effects that seem to arise from vaccinations. Some homoeopaths give it quite routinely for this purpose. In case of ailments following vaccination, where any of the thuja features noted above are present, it may be given with some confidence.

TUBERCULINUM, tub

Remedy source: see nosodes, p. 197. See also note on varieties below.

Main uses

Tuberculinum is a familiar constitutional type and the most widely used of the major nosodes. It is sometimes given in short-term conditions, mostly of the chest.

Characteristics

Tuberculinum individuals feel restless and dissatisfied. They are sensitive, but their feelings are more aesthetic than really emotional. They are gregarious, but do not form deep attachments to anyone or anything. The only emotion they feel strongly and consistently is a kind of discontent, an inner urge to experience and explore. A desire to travel is the best-known feature of the tuberculinum mind. It is this combination of being driven to seek fulfilment, together with an odd lack of emotional involvement, that seems to characterise the type.

It is a common remedy in children. Without the ability to express themselves in sophisticated ways, or the means to indulge the urge to travel and experiment, they can become very irritable. Often they are bright, even precocious, but with a capacity for horrible moods, in which they can be actually violent and destructive. In the various degrees of hyperactivity and tantrums in children, tuberculinum is one of the most important remedies.

In the more independent adults the temper tantrums are less prominent. They travel, they indulge, they put down few roots. They can have a mean temper, often related to their impatience to move on quickly, and unrestrained by emotional warmth. But adults are rarely actually violent. An interesting feature of the tuberculinum mind, highly suggestive of what remains unintegrated within them, is a common fear of dogs and, particularly in children, cats.

Physical tendencies and weak points
Physically, both children and adults are usually long and lean, even though they have a big appetite. Bones and skin are fine. Pressure around the waistband makes them very uncomfortable. Thick eyelashes and hair along the spine are common in the children. Typically, they have a strong liking for milk, meats like salami, and bananas. They do not tolerate the cold well, but have a strong need for the open air.

The weak point is mostly the chest. All kinds of respiratory conditions may require tuberculinum. Poor development, allergies and menstrual troubles are also common.

The tubercular taint
Like the other nosodes tuberculinum is sometimes of great benefit to individuals who display a tubercular 'taint', without all the symptoms noted above. In such cases it could be just stubborn chest complaints and a distant family history of tuberculosis, combined with the fact that other remedies were helping little, that indicates the need for tuberculinum, after which other remedies will resume their good work.

Varieties of tuberculinum and bacillinum

There are several strains of tuberculinum in general use. A bovine (cattle) sample (tuberculinum bovinum, tub bov) has been widely used. So too has a human sample, known as tuberculinum koch (tub koch), after the doctor who prepared it. A remedy called bacillinum was prepared from the sputum of a human tuberculosis sufferer. The symptoms of these nosodes are difficult to distinguish in practice. References in this book are to tub koch unless otherwise indicated.

URTICA URENS, urtica, urt-u

Remedy source: plant—stinging nettle.

Main uses

The juice and potentised forms of this very familiar plant are both quite widely used, for a variety of short-term problems. No personality profile has been observed, and the remedy is often given in situations where no clear psychological element is present in the case.

Burns. Locally and internally for the itching and pain of minor burns, including sunburn.

Rashes. Especially those that look like the effects of stinging nettles. Hives, urticaria. All sorts of itchy, blistered skin eruptions. Allergic reactions.

Lactation. Both to increase and dry up the flow of milk in nursing mothers.

Gout. For the acute attacks.

VERATRUM ALBUM, verat alb, verat

Remedy source: plant—white hellebore.

Main uses

This remedy is used for severe cases of collapse and vomiting and diarrhoea, occasionally in temperate climates, and more commonly in tropical ones. A constitutional type has also been described.

Specific conditions
Fever or collapse. The patient is very cold, blue, and covered in cold sweat. The gastric conditions are accompanied by intense cramping pains and great thirst. Profuse vomiting and diarrhoea simultaneously are very characteristic.

Constitutional type

This type is not very common, but distinctive enough to be familiar. The outstanding characteristic of veratrum people is intense insecurity about their place in the world. In response they become ambitious, although often it is just the trappings of success and status that they need to be satisfied. They may develop very strong views, and cannot imagine how they could be reconciled to those who think differently. There is often a strong religious element in their feelings. At the heart of it all is the insecurity about their personal position, and the remedy may be needed by the jealous siblings of younger children.

Homoeopathic Resources

Australia

Representative organisation with information on where to contact a homoeopath
Australian Homoeopathic Association, 65 Broseley Road, Toowong, Queensland 4066.
Tel: 07 3870 5765. Fax: 07 3371 7245. email:georgec@uq.net.au

Pharmacies and suppliers of homoeopathic medicines
Brauer Biotherapies, 1 Para Road, Tanunda, SA 5352.
Tel: 08 85632932

Colleges
The Sydney College of Homoeopathic Medicine, PO Box 448, Leichhardt, Sydney, NSW 2040.
Tel: 02 9564 6731

Victorian College of Classical Homoeopathy, Suite 3A, 574 Whitehorse Road, Mitcham, Victoria 3132.
Tel: 03 9873 0567

Canada

Representative organisation with information on where to contact a homoeopath
National United Professional Association of Trained Homoeopaths (Canada), 1445 St Joseph Boulevard, Gloucester, Ontario, K1C 7K9.
Tel: (613) 830-4759. rudi@web.net

Pharmacies and suppliers of homoeopathic medicines
Boiron Canada, 816 Guimond Boulevard, Longueil, Montreal, Quebec, J4G 1T5.
Tel: (514) 442-2066. Fax: (514) 442-9079

Stafford Pharmacy and Home Healthcare, 1475 St Edward Boulevard North, Lethbridge, Alberta, T1H 2P9.
Tel: (403) 320-6500

Colleges
The Canadian Academy of Homoeopathy, 203–3044 Bloor Street W, Toronto, Ontario, M8X 2Y8.
Tel: (416) 503-4003. Enquiries on course content: Tel: (416) 425-4829

School of Homoeopathy, Devon (North American Flexible Learning Program), 4 Oakvale Place SW, Calgary, Alberta, T2V 1H4.
Tel: (403) 281-7976

Homoeopathic College of Canada, 280 Eglinton Avenue East, Toronto, Ontario, M4P 1L4.
Tel: (416) 481–8816. Toll free: 1-888-DR-HOMEO (374-6636). info@homoeopathy.edu

Toronto School of Homoeopathic Medicine (TSHM), 17 Yorkville Avenue, Toronto, Ontario, M4W 1L1.
Tel: (416) 966-2350. Toll-free: 800-572-6001

New Zealand

Representative organisation with information on where to contact a homoeopath
New Zealand Council of Homoeopaths, PO Box 51-195, Tawa.
Tel: 04 232 7942. email: jwinston@actrix.gen.nz

Pharmacies and suppliers of homoeopathic medicines
Simillimum Homoeopathic Pharmacy, 20 Panama Street, Wellington.
Tel: 0800 ARNICA (276 422) or 04 499 9242. orders@arnica.co.nz

Selene Homoeopathics, PO Box 2456, Tauranga.
Tel: 07 578 3635

Lincoln Mall Pharmacy, 254 Lincoln Road, Henderson.
Tel: 09 838 8576

Weleda (NZ) Ltd, Peak Road, Hastings.
Tel: 06 877 7394

Colleges
Auckland College of Classical Homoeopathy, PO Box 19502, Auckland.
Tel: 09 828 9700

Bay of Plenty College of Homoeopathy, PO Box 784 Tauranga.
Tel: 0-25-467 133

Wellington College of Homoeopathy, 99 Main Road, Tawa, Wellington.
Tel: 04 232 7942

South Africa

Representative organisation with information on where to contact a homoeopath
Homoeopathic Association of South Africa, PO Box 87490, Houghton 2041.
Tel: 011 453 6830

Pharmacies and suppliers of homoeopathic medicines
A. Whites Homoeopathic Pharmacy, 77 Plein Street, Cape Town.
Tel: 021 465 3382

Weleda Pharmacy, PO Box 7297, Johannesburg 2000.
Tel: 011 333 1571. email: paul.booyse@pixie.co.za

Pharma Natura, PO Box 86, Howard Place 7450, Cape Town.
Tel: 021 555 1144

W. Last Pharmacy, PO Box 407, Johannesburg 2000.
Tel: 011 680 5580 or 021 47 9895

Colleges
Department of Homoeopathy, Technikon Natal, Box 953, 4000 Durban.
Tel: 031 204 2542

School of Homoeopathy, Teknikon Witwatersrand, Faculty of Health and Biotechnology, Box 17011, Doornfontein 2028.
Tel: 011 406 2450

United Kingdom

Representative organisations with information on where to contact a homoeopath
The Society of Homoeopaths, 4a Artizan Road, Northampton NN1 4HU.
Tel: 01604 622622

The Faculty of Homoeopathy, 15 Clerkenwell Close, London EC1R 0AA.
Tel: 020 7566 7810/5

Pharmacies and suppliers of homoeopathic medicines
Ainsworths Homoeopathic Pharmacy, 36 New Cavendish Street, London W1M 7LH.
Tel: 0171 935 5330

Freemans Homoeopathic Pharmacy, 20 Main Street, Busby, Glasgow G76 8DU.
Tel: 0141 644 1165

Helios Homoeopathic Pharmacy, 97 Camden Road, Tunbridge Wells, Kent TN1 2QR.
Tel: 01892 537 254

Nelsons Homoeopathic Pharmacy, 73 Duke Street, London W1M 6BY.
Tel: 0171 629 3118

Colleges
The Faculty of Homoeopathy (as above).
Runs courses in homoeopathy for doctors of medicine.

The Society of Homoeopaths (as above).
Keeps a list of several colleges running courses which it recognises as leading to admission to its register of qualified homoeopaths.

United States

Representative organisations with information on where to contact a homoeopath
The National Center for Homoeopathy, 801 North Fairfax Street, Suite 306, Alexandria, VA 22314.
Tel: (703) 548-7790

Homoeopathic Academy of Naturopathic Physicians, PO Box 12488, Portland, OR 97212.
Tel: 503 795–0579

North American Society of Homoeopaths, 122 East Pike Street, Suite 1122, Seattle, WA 98122.
Tel: 206 720 7000. www.homoeopathy.org

Pharmacies and suppliers of homoeopathic remedies
Boericke and Tafel Inc, 2381 Circadian Way, Santa Rosa, CA 95407.
Tel: (707) 571-8202

Boiron-Bornemann Inc, Box 449, 6 Campus Avenue, Building A, Newtown Square, PA 19073.
Tel: (800)BLU-TUBE

Boiron-Bornemann Inc, 98c W Cochran Street, Simi Valley, CA 93065.
Tel: (800) 258-8823

Dolisos America Inc, 3014 Rigel Avenue, Las Vegas, NV 89102.
Tel: 1-800–DOLISOS (800) 365-4767

Standard Homoeopathic Company, PO Box 61067, 204-210 W 131st Street, Los Angeles, CA 90061.
Tel: (800) 624-9659

Washington Homoeopathic Products Inc, 4914 Del Ray Avenue, Bethesda, MD 20814.
Tel: (800) 336-1695 (orders). (304) 258-2541 (business, information)

Weleda Pharmacy, Inc, 841 S Main Street, Chestnut Ridge, New York 10977.
Tel: (914) 352-6165

Colleges
The National Center for Homoeopathy (as above).

Information on the Internet

For all countries, as well as the sites and email addresses noted above, a lot of information is available on the internet. A good place to start is www.homoeopathyhome.com

INDEX